D1430882

BECOME A
CONSCIOUSNESS
ATHLETE

A STEP BY STEP PROGRAM TO HEIGHTEN
CONSCIOUSNESS FOR DAILY HAPPINESS

BETHANY GONYEA, MS

NUMINOUS

Quantum Health Solutions

Become A Consciousness Athlete
A Step By Step Program To Heighten Consciousness For Daily Happiness
Copyright © 2021 by Bethany A. Gonyea, MS
Digital ISBN: 978-1-7364149-5-8

DEDICATION

To my Darling Daughters

I delayed having children until later in life because I wanted to teach you things I did not know as a young woman. More than teaching you just how to brush your teeth and your ABC's, I wanted to teach you to sustain the heart of a poet, the sight of a visionary, and the spirit of a child.
It was not until I finished this book that I realized how much you inspired me to write it.
You are my greatest teachers.
I hope that I have lived as a model of this work for you.
I love you more than you will ever know.

Mom

INTRODUCTION

What if you had the power to change your negative emotional states on demand? What if you could pivot out of depression without consuming food, alcohol, or drugs, or traveling back in time to change the past? How would it feel to be buoyantly happy for "no good reason"?

You may say, "Well, that would be great, but it isn't possible. I feel the way I feel because of all the things that have gone wrong in my life. I would be happier if A happened, B didn't happen, and if I had more of C. I understand. You might have been happier if A happened, B didn't happen, and you had more of C, but how much of that can you change? Probably, you can't change these circumstances, which is why you need to know that you have the power to be buoyantly happy at this moment, regardless of the tragedies you have faced in your life.

Does that sound impossible? I can assure you, it isn't. This book will show you how happiness is merely a state of being in your body's nervous system and energy field, independent of your outer circumstances. If you want to be happy badly enough, you simply need to train your body's nervous system to sustain heightened states of well-being. I understand that this process may seem vague, but it isn't. It follows the exact same process that an athlete uses to train the body to play sports, or a musician uses to perform music. Using the mind-body skills in this book, you will learn how to become physically rooted in an empowered stance of well-being. A stance that enables you to feel whole and complete, regardless of your external circumstances.

Happiness researchers have discovered that external factors are only responsible for 10% of our happiness levels. Take a moment to think about that fact. Our internal happiness levels are influenced by only 10% by our life situations. The remaining 90% of factors affecting our happiness are determined by our inner world, including our genes, behavior choices, and perceptions. Basically, how we feel on the inside significantly affects how we perceive external factors. If we change how we feel on the inside, it changes how we perceive external circumstances. Learning how to change how we feel, not how we think, offers us the enormous latitude to dramatically improve our lives" quality.

Many of us have undergone talk therapy to help us understand our inner world. We have cultivated self-awareness, explored complicated relationships, and learned how our family of origin influences our behaviors. These experiences are beneficial, but often talk therapy can stop us just short of happiness. By undergoing treatment, we may learn why we tend toward certain destructive behaviors, but this knowledge may have little impact. I once heard a therapist say, "As a social worker, I am really good at helping clients understand why they drink, but I am ineffective at inspiring them not to drink." This social worker acknowledges that merely changing our reasoning or thinking patterns often does not make us happier. So, if reasoning ourselves into more joyful spaces will not make us happier, then what will?

How we experience the external world is dramatically influenced by our state of being, which has everything to do with how we feel, both physically and emotionally, instead of what we are thinking. Happiness can seem elusive, but only because most of us have not been trained in managing our body's nervous system and energy fields. When we change how we feel on the inside of the body, we significantly alter our response patterns.

Let me give you an example. Have you ever been

drifting to sleep at night, and suddenly a troubling topic enters your mind? It causes agitation, and you find yourself unable to sleep. Then, you are surprised after waking the following morning to find that it does not bother you nearly as much when you review the same subject. That is because, at the end of a long day, your body is tired and has fewer energetic resources to tackle thorny problems. In the morning, when you are well-rested, the issue does not loom so large. You have more energetic resources. Being "hangry" is the same idea. When we are hungry, situations annoy us more, and we tend to become angrier than if we weren't hungry.

For the past two decades, we have seen an explosion of happiness books, suggesting that adopting behaviors such as journaling, random acts of kindness, or listing things you are grateful for each day will boost mood. These mood-enhancers can work nicely. However, this book addresses how to prime your body and mind to orient your state of being to happiness, so you actually want to do these life-affirming behaviors. The difference is that this book will teach you how to create an internal environment that enables you to choose these behaviors as a natural extension of the happiness you already feel, not because you believe that doing them will make you feel happier.

I am not trying to be pedantic. I am talking about

a critically different skill set: the "pre-existing condition" for engaging in more healthy, mood-enhancing behaviors instead of just ritualistically performing them with the hope they might make you happier. We all know what we "should" do to feel better in life, right? Exercise, eat right, watch less Netflix, work on our relationships more. But do we actually follow through with these behaviors that will make us happier? If not, why not? I suggest we don't do what we know would make us happy because our state of being is not calibrated correctly to want to be happy.

This pre-existing condition for happiness is how we are "seated" or poised in our body's nervous system. Suppose we are not poised correctly in our nervous system to sustain happiness. In that case, we could win millions in the lottery, and our mood would still eventually deflate to our nervous system's baseline of unhappiness before winning the lottery.

I have been unceasingly fascinated with how to focus our minds on lifting sour moods for over two decades. This skill is so personally and physically experiential; I can't convey this work's power through only concepts and words: you will need to cultivate this exquisite state of being through practicing the six mind-body explorations that accompany this book. These explorations teach you how to focus your mind like a laser in the body to release negativity with precision. I am personally a big fan of instant healthy gratification, so I have designed these explorations to help you experience a rapid, pleasant shift in your orientation to your world around you. Once you recognize how quickly you can change your state of being, you will never feel limited to influence your mood again. I have seen this work transform thousands of lives. I want you to have these powerful experiences that are, literally, located underneath your nose!

By experiencing the six mind-body explorations, you will quickly learn that we don't experience happiness in our minds. We experience pleasure in our bodies! Does that shift your understanding a bit? When we change how we feel on the inside of our bodies, we drastically change how we feel about the world outside our bodies. When our bodies feel at ease, we feel at ease. When our bodies are "happier," we are happier. Feelings of happiness do not occur in our minds—they happen in our bodies. When we feel happy, our body is secreting a cascade of chemicals, especially dopamine, that provide the emotion of happiness.

I wrote this book to share what I have learned about how to invoke the cascade of positive chemicals in our bodies, to activate happiness hormones in any circumstance. The skills offered in this book have been honed from teaching cutting-edge biofeedback skills for over twenty-five years. I cherry-picked the best skills to ensure your state of being will be enhanced. I teach only what I have tested myself and have seen to be successful with others, and I have incredibly high standards.

I trained my body to hold buoyant states in the most challenging circumstances, including facing the death of family members, unknown financial and family outcomes, and pursuing pioneering professional goals—that have never before been accomplished. These skills have worked, but not for me alone. They have also been useful for thousands of people I have worked with over the years, who have learned how to increase awareness in their bodies and foster more buoyant states of well-being, even during uncertain times. In recent years, I have begun to refer to my students and myself as "Consciousness or Happiness Athletes" because we are creating the endurance in our nervous systems to hold buoyant emotional states for extended periods of time. I love having company on this journey! In light of the positive results I've witnessed in myself and others, I believe this information is too useful and world-changing to keep to myself.

I have chosen the word "athlete" to reflect this process of training for a specific reason. This book offers you the skills to train your nervous system to sustain happiness; the way athletes condition their bodies to perform sports well. Musicians are similar to athletes in that they have to maintain an internal physical poise to play their instruments during performances. What if you practiced tuning your body to create beautiful, ambient music within yourself? With proper training, you are capable of "changing your state" into buoyant happiness at will. You are that powerful!

Practicing to maintain a state of joy and satisfaction in life, regardless of life's challenges, is one of the most profound gifts you could ever give yourself. If you learn these skills now, then one day, on your deathbed, you will rest in a deep satisfaction that you were so "present and accounted for" in life, that you did not miss your opportunity to love, dance, or be free at any moment. You will face the end of your life, knowing that you "showed up" in this life, embracing every moment for what it had to offer you, and making the world better by your presence. Your ability to be available and free within your own body gave you the resilience to press on when life knocked you down, and to feel the joy of discovery as you picked yourself back up. You learned the game of life, and you learned how to play it well! If you master this book's skills you will approach death with the same open heart for adventure that enables you to savor your life now.

After twenty-five years of teaching people how to change their states at will, I know this exquisite state of being is not only possible but is your birthright. I have been humbled time and again by the privilege of witnessing transformations within minutes. People under the tyranny of profound loss finally feel a break from grief. An annoying, persistent headache finally gets relieved. A nagging problem suddenly feels manageable. Living a life without the owner's manual to your nervous system is one of the greatest human tragedies.

I believe that every person should know their birthright to feel buoyant. I created my non-profit NUMINOUS, and its outreach program, *the Global Peaceful Cities Project,* to teach everyday people how to access the beauty within them. However, this book will take you further than I can guide through our public peace meditation research studies. This book outlines the fundamental, core skills covered in our popular course, The Consciousness Athlete Program. In the mind-body explorations accompanying this book, I have embedded the most potent mind-body skills that I have honed and taught during my twenty-five years in the field of biofeedback, which is the art, and science of using the mind to positively influence the body.

While teaching biofeedback, I've had a persistent, compelling daydream, which appears like this: I imagine an infant entering this world, and after she takes her first breath, an Angel descends and whispers in her ear,

Hey, Beautiful, I thought you might like to know you were born with a body that has a nervous system. Facing this life's inevitable struggles will be extremely challenging if you don't learn how to toggle your nervous system from negativity into well-being. This lack of skill may seriously thwart your progress through depression, endless rumination, or substance abuse. But if you do learn how to come into command of your nervous system, to lead it into heightened states of well-being, you will ride through life's endless difficulties with consistent ease and grace. At times, you may even become captivated by wonder and awe along the way.

This daydream recurs when I witness people enduring hardship. Hearing them share their deepest conflicts, dormant dreams, and daily struggles, I often wish I could instantly impart my knowledge into their nervous system. I want to help others dramatically accelerate through the steep learning curve I had. This book is my attempt to help you expedite your journey to happiness. There is absolutely no reason to wait!

Furthermore, this work is an equal opportunity game-changer. No one can be left behind because we will be training your nervous system, and every human being has one. I have pioneered mindfulness biofeedback programs in dozens of schools, mostly inner-city schools of underserved families. These students demonstrate these skills go a very long way, helping individuals compensate for inequities. By learning how to come into command of their nervous systems, students become amazingly resilient, even in the face of enormous loss.

For example, before practicing meditation, I often ask the students, "how are you feeling now?" The answers I receive are often "annoyed," "bored," "restless," "angry," "depressed." Then, after our skilled biofeedback mind-body explorations, I ask them, How do you feel now? Their answers may range from "excited," to "happy," "calm," "content," and "peaceful." Then, I say in an astonished tone, to let them know how impressive their state change really is:

Do you realize how amazing it is that you know how to use your mind as a superpower to change your mood at will? One minute you are angry, depressed, and bored, and three minutes later, you are happy, light, and peaceful? Do you know that most grown-ups don't know how to change their states like that, which is why you may see them overdo drugs and alcohol? Adults do those things because they are trying to change their internal state. You will never have to take recreational drugs, or drink alcohol to excess because you have already learned how to change your internal states without giving your power over to food, drugs, or substances. Now, do you now understand how powerful you are?

We were born to feel fabulous. We have opiate receptors throughout our entire body; our brains and bodies are equipped to "get high" and feel pleasure without drugs or alcohol. We can maintain buoyant states in the body if we do not override them with racing thoughts, resentful mental cul-de-sacs, and relentless attachments to unhealthy behaviors. Kids can be our teachers of this phenomenon. They can have a bad experience, and often they will go out to play relatively soon afterward. As adults, we have developed poor coping habits, such as posting our misery on social media, going out for caffeine, sugar, or alcohol with friends to tell them how bad our luck is, and choosing self-sabotaging behaviors that only make us feel worse about our defeats.

When I look into a classroom after leading a mind-body exploration and observe how, within mere minutes, the dull eyes of students have turned bright; their sluggish postures have become erect; and their furrowed brows have become smooth; I feel blessed yet again to be a teacher of peace! As teachers and students recognize me walking through school halls, they remember the skills I teach. I see them suddenly taking a deep breath. Often they will ask, "Are you coming to our room today?" with positive anticipation because they remember the good feelings this work brings them.

I did not always have this resilient disposition. I did not always "fall up." My father was a raving alcoholic who left when I was three. I was raised by my mom, a food-addicted religious zealot, who suffered global depressions for months at a time. When I first started my healing journey, uninformed counselors would try to coax me to access more pleasant memories by asking me to remember happy childhood experiences. This question actually made me feel worse because I would wrack my brain, trying to think of positive moments to resource. I eventually started making up positive memories to give myself a reference point.

Based on my genetic and personal history, it was not in my genes to write a book on enduring happiness! I only tell this story because I don't want to sound glib. I don't want you to say to yourself, "Well, it is easy for her. She has not had the losses I have." A dark childhood brings challenges as an adult that I would not wish on anyone. But, ironically, I often feel that I am happy because of those harrowing experiences. I have been blessed to be in a professional field that offered powerful rudimentary skills to help me successfully ride through my losses. I built on those skills persistently to be sure I experience what psychologists call post-traumatic growth, which occurs when people become happier after tragic losses. When we learn how to use suffering to promote positive growth constructively, there is no limit on our happiness.

Living as a Consciousness Athlete means facing your life with a set of skills that empower you to experience an increase in satisfaction from any challenge. I use every conflict I face as an opportunity, a chance to practice honing my ability to maintain well-being in my body for extended periods. I utilize the mind-body skills offered in this book to stabilize my nervous system and relax under pressure. These skills help me rebound so that I feel stronger, more poised, and open to even more good feelings after the conflict is resolved. The cumulative benefits of this work over time have conditioned my body to maintain well-being, which causes my happiness baseline to rise continuously. These benefits inspire me to fall more in love with this work every day.

But this elevation in "resting happiness" didn't happen because, during my woes, I collapsed into binge-watching Netflix while eating a pint of Ben and Jerry's. My joy increased because I chose to face my pain by applying the tools I share in this book. I trained my nervous system like athletes train their bodies. Through pleasant exploration, I learned I have far greater control over my emotions, addictions, behaviors, and pleasures than I have ever been taught.

Through these skills, I tweaked my inner world to feel brighter each day by applying these skills during simple daily activities. I became happier because of my traumas, not despite them.

In this book, I share the mind-body biofeedback skills to help you develop a fundamental mastery of your mind and body. I hope to inspire a lifelong passion for applying these skills so that you live an empowered life in real life. I want to offer you the perspective to face each day knowing that you have a powerful context from which you can meet your challenges and win. These skills can make the difference between feeling like you are traveling aimlessly in life versus walking with great dignity, nobility, and purpose. I know I will use these skills until the day I die, and while I am dying: for the skills we need to die exceptionally well are the same skills we need to live exceptionally well. I have observed people struggling at the end of life because they had no inner navigation as their external body failed. Tragically, this caused them additional anguish and pain during their final days. I don't wish that for you. Paradoxically, when you learn these skills to live better, you face death with greater ease and poise, as well.

To help you understand just how vital this work is in the context of your whole life, you need to know that the verdict on happiness is out! Happy people perform better in all areas of life. Their marriages are more content, and so are their children. Research has even shown that happy people live an average of 7-9 years longer! Another reason to take your happiness seriously is that it benefits the people around you as well. Think about it: how important is it for a parent to be happy? How important is it for a teacher to be happy? I promise you that you want both your lawyer and your doctor to be happy! You don't want to be under the professional direction of any unhappy person. Happiness research has demonstrated that happier people are more successful in all areas of life. Paradoxically, when we work to fill our well of happiness, we become less self-involved, so we are more available to serve others.

To accelerate this learning, you will need to be sure to practice the mind-body audio explorations included in this book. The good news is that you will gain instant gratification if you commit to this work. This work has to work. If you apply it, it can't not work! Think of it this way: you can't repetitively lift weights at a gym and not get more strong. Right? That would be impossible. You can't do this work and not increase your capacity for happiness because that would be impossible as well. We all want to feel better, and within minutes of starting the mind-body explorations that accompany this book, you will already be changing your state of being.

You will soon understand why words can teach

very little in this realm. People need profound experiences in their nervous system to fully master this work. The skill-building explorations included in this book will build internal skills, mastery, and stamina. Please practice these mind-body audio explorations in the order they are presented to establish fundamental skills first before attempting the more advanced skills. If you choose to only to read this book, you will be learning only a fraction of the information needed to become a Consciousness Athlete.

Our culture has a fascination with exposure to words and memes as a substitute for learning or experience. This cognitive information preference is partially responsible for the skyrocketing incidences of anxiety medication use, rampant substance abuse, and obesity statistics. These unhealthy behaviors are merely attempts to self-soothe. Most of us were not taught how to self-soothe in healthy ways. In our frantic content-driven culture, we desperately need tools to unburden ourselves. Please be sure to give yourself the gift of these mind-body skill explorations, so this information can make the lasting impact I know it can have in your life. No one can do this work but you, but I promise you I will make the work itself enjoyable!

I am a highly-skilled teacher with years of gritty experience working with people to alter their nervous systems. I've worked with all age groups, from infants to one hundred-year-olds, including many subgroups such as police, law students, inmates, and elementary to college students. Still, I can't help you if you don't value your happiness enough to take the time to skillfully dive within yourself and come into mastery of your own nervous system. No one can ever do that for you. Only you can. My intention for writing this book is to inspire you to take this personal, intimate journey. If you accept this journey, I offer you a 100% guarantee that you will find yourself far more fascinating than you ever realized. You will even recover an enchantment with life that you may feel you've been missing.

Each mind-body skill building exploration has a suggested practice schedule for minimal competency. Your nervous system needs both routine and novelty for it to stay engaged with learning. You will need to repeatedly practice each mind-body exploration about five times because the first time you listen, will so entertain you with the novel task, you won't truly grasp the learning. I suggest that you repeat each exploration five times. You may find that some of these explorations will speak to you more than others, and you will want to return to some explorations more than others. If so, that is perfect. Each mind-body skill building exploration balances your nervous system in a specific way. If you prefer one of them, it means that it enhances the functioning of the unique way your nervous system is wired.

After gaining some necessary mastery over our physical nervous system, we will learn to explore what I call subtle energy biofeedback. You will learn to come into greater command of the bioelectric life force traveling through and around the circuits in your body, often referred to as the acupuncture meridian system. As we learn to become still in the body, we learn to experience an exquisite awareness, which dramatically expands our perceptions. This expansion of awareness gives us keys to a much more extensive range of possibilities for our lives. At this point in your learning, you may be surprised and delighted to realize this work is a lifelong discovery process, one that only gets better with additional time and effort.

After finishing the mind-body explorations in this book, you have the opportunity to put your new mind-body skills effortlessly into service for others, which will simultaneously increase your happiness even more. It is common for people who have undergone a healing path to have a strong desire to share their discoveries with others. The information in this book will allow you to make a powerful change outside in the world from the privacy of your own home. To allow people an opportunity to share their new skills in a meaningful, tangible manner, I created the *Global Peaceful Cities Project*, an outreach of my non-profit, NUMINOUS. I invite you to become part of our Collective Meditation Peace Corps, where we measure how groups of Consciousness Athletes positively influence the world by sending intentions for peace to geographic areas. To date, we have performed two research studies, demonstrating that our intentions for peace in the world have already achieved real-world impact. We will talk more about this later, but if you want a sneak peek, please visit PeacefulCities.org.

Are you ready to be truly happy? Are you ready to cultivate the exquisite state of well-being that is well within your reach? Then let's keep going. Other Consciousness Athletes are waiting to hear from you! You will have the opportunity to share your deepest longings for peace in a community that will support you in some of the rarest, most meaningful ways possible.

CHAPTER 1 - YOUR MIND HAS IMPACT—SO BE CAREFUL WITH IT!

What if we all cultivated a profound respect for our mind and the thoughts it provides? What if we stopped overlooking our thoughts as impotent and started seeing them as the powerful, even formidable, creative force they actually are?

I have cultivated a profound respect for thought during the last twenty-five years because I have witnessed the impact thoughts have on our bodies in real-time while observing measurements biofeedback instrumentation. Biofeedback is the art and science of teaching people how to use their minds to influence the body positively. I do this by connecting people's bodies to an instrument that measures different physical processes, such as blood pressure, heart rate, muscle tension, or perspiration. When the client's mind flickers in a meaningful manner, the body always mimics the internal change of thoughts, evidenced by measurable changes in the biofeedback readings. Your thoughts command that much power!

Your thoughts can even command your entire nervous system. For instance, your thoughts can activate your body to create complex chemical cocktails, capable of leading your body toward disease or health, depression or bliss, toward complete chaos or total mastery. Through biofeedback training, I teach people how to harness the power of their thoughts to influence the body in palpable ways positively. This training enables clients to lower their blood pressure, eliminate migraine headaches, or even increase blood flow to their hands and feet, which is especially helpful for people who suffer from Raynaud's syndrome. Everyone is this powerful after they have learned how to focus their minds with discipline.

Biofeedback instruments offer us the power to see the immediate impact of thoughts on our bodies in "real-time." For instance, when I connect people to a galvanic skin response (GSR) biofeedback instrument, which measures changes in sweat gland activity in the fingers, they often look incredulous when they hear the device emit an annoying squeal as they ruminate upon stressful thoughts. They are equally perplexed when the pitch lowers as they contemplate more serene topics. Often, during my biofeedback presentations, I nudge the person who is on stage demonstrating the GSR with me, asking them in front of the large group to "tell us three difficult situations in your life, right now, that are making you feel raw." Before I even finish the sentence, the GSR pitch dramatically skyrockets, and the audience starts to chuckle. The mere thought of specific stressors triggers greater sweat in the body, making the GSR register stark changes. Then I often comment, "You don't have to tell us what your challenges are. Your body has already told us. But see if you can list three the three stressors only in your mind." The audience becomes intrigued because as the person mentally reviews each stressor, it is apparent when the person thinks of a new one after the instrument immediately responds. Turning to the audience, I ask, "Are you starting to understand how your body eavesdrops on everything you think?"

Through biofeedback training, people gain a deep respect for the power of their thoughts on their bodies. They start becoming more discerning about which ideas are worth exploring and which thoughts need to be left behind permanently. For years, I have been encouraging people to "feel their mental thoughts." When I ask clients to do this, it means that I am asking them to frequently stop as they ruminate on topics and take a moment to learn how each thought feels in the body. As we slow down our racing thinking, we have the opportunity to cultivate a profound awareness of our mind-body connection, that will warn us when we are spiraling into anxiety, unhealthy addictive patterns, and disempowering self-sabotage. The more we remain anchored in the body and become aware of our thoughts' negative consequences, the harder it becomes for us to fool ourselves into perpetuating unhealthy patterns.

In private sessions, I ask clients to discuss troubling challenges in their lives and observe how the pitch of the galvanic skin response changes. As they tell me about their problematic job situation or their challenging relationship, the pitch rises. I explain to them that even though they are not at their job or with their partner, their nervous system responds as if they are. I then teach them how to keep the pitch low as they review these problematic situations in their lives.

The first skill I teach people is how to anchor their minds in their bodies while discussing difficult topics. I do this by having them lie on my massage table and focus their minds while remaining aware of specific places in their bodies. I remind them to listen and determine how the pitch changes. For instance, I have them place their hand on their torso and become aware of their hand's heat on their abdomen. I ask them to anchor their mind's awareness under their thumb first, then under their index finger, middle finger, ring finger, and pinky. I guide them to imagine that their awareness is "swimming around" inside their body, similar to a scuba diver swimming in deep water. They are asked to "dive" their awareness deep into their body, and feel the fleshy portion of each finger from "inside" of their torso.

As people attempt to do this, the GSR pitch often wavers as their minds flicker, indicating how often our ability to hold our minds still is compromised. Most people do not have this basic level of mental discipline, especially in our video-gaming, social media, and Netflix culture, which is why so many of us needlessly suffer. Our society has become comfortable, allowing ourselves to be passively entertained by external stimuli for a large portion of our lives. Unfortunately, along with this increase in entertainment, we simultaneously lost some of our ability to direct ourselves. The GSR will reveal any weakness in this area, immediately and precisely. As the mind flits in and out of the body, the GSR mirrors the fluctuation of internal instability.

Eventually, most clients can establish at least a modicum of control over anchoring their minds to their abdomen, which means they have gained enough mastery to proceed with our exploration. We move their awareness down to their right hip next. I ask permission to hold my hand at the side of their right hip, and ask them to "touch my hand with your mind." As their awareness dives deeper in their body, the GSR pitch descends similarly, mimicking their more significant descent of awareness into their body. Next, I place my hand on the back of their right knee and invite them to anchor their mind there again, asking them to "touch my hand with your mind." We soon move their mind's awareness to their ankle and the bottom of their foot. Each time they shift their consciousness lower in their body, the pitch of the GSR lowers. I make sure to help them notice: each time they focus their awareness more downward in their body; the GSR reflects the shift as the pitch falls as well.

After their mind is stabilized enough in their own body, I ask them to recall any situations that are causing them stress. Immediately, the GSR pitch rises. But then I ask them to remain anchored in the body as they review their challenges. Their mind often wants to immediately vacate the body as they get more immersed in discussing their challenges. I gently encourage them to remain anchored in the body while striving to keep the GSR pitch low. Most people experience what I call a "mental tongue twister."

Do you remember trying to say tongue twisters when you were a child? Tongue twisters are a sequence of words or sounds, typically alliterative, difficult to pronounce quickly and correctly. For example, "tie twine to three tree twigs". Easy enough when you read it, but try saying it out loud several times in a row. It can be very frustrating. It is a very similar internal feeling of frustration for most people, trying to remain anchored in their body while reviewing their stressors. An undisciplined mind will run wild. Often the person demonstrating the GSR will look like a picture of peace outwardly, but when I ask them if it was easy to keep the pitch low, they say something like, "hell no!" When I ask, "Did you feel like you were fighting for your life to keep the pitch down?" they laugh wholeheartedly and say, "Yes!"

Having done hundreds of these demonstrations over the last twenty-five years, I've witnessed how this one experience can dramatically change people's lives. Later on, participants love to share how pivotal it was to be that person on stage, demonstrating the GSR. In such a short time, they learned a powerful, fundamental truth about their mind's "focus" and realized that where their mind lands impact every aspect of their lives. Many of these people have shared with me that this one experience internally shifted them permanently for life. In the first mind-body audio exploration accompanying this book, I will help you experience the power of this truth deep within you. Tragically, most of us have been taught to overlook this truth our entire lives, and yet it influences all of our perceptions and experiences.

To help you learn this concept through contrast, in the first mind-body audio exploration, you will learn how to anchor your mind in your body . . . on only one side of your body! The contrast of being present in only one side of the body, compared to being "absent" on the other side, will teach you more than any words I can write. I will take you on a journey where you will distinctly feel the considerable difference between where your mind is anchored in the body and where it is not. People learn that their minds can be so impactful, that they find their bodies even leaning to one side! I offer this exploration, because I am not asking anyone to take my word for anything I say. I want them to have the opportunity to experience it for themselves. Then I ask, "From which side of the body would you prefer to live your life?" People inevitably answer that it is the side where their mind is now anchored.

Because people immediately understand that they have only scratched the surface of something much more significant, I ask another provocative question: "If you would prefer living from the state of consciousness of being present in the side of your body that you are now anchored, after only seven minutes of this experience, how much more might you prefer to live from that space after practicing this state of consciousness for seven days? What if every day you learned to be present in the body a little bit more? How different would you feel in thirty days?" People often don't respond, right away as they feel into that state of consciousness which reveals wisdom beyond words. They realize they have not been "in their body" for years and wonder how different life would be if they were more present.

We have become a culture that is frightened to feel our bodies, which is why we experience profuse suffering through anxiety disorders, substance abuse, obesity issues, insomnia, and chronic, unexplained pain. Feeling emotions and sensations has become frightening for a culture that lives in their head and beyond. This work trains us in a mental-physical discipline to enhance our state of being because the body does not lie. The body will tell you if you are feeling apathetic, terrified or overwhelmed. We may look calm, but our bodies reveal the raw truth when we are connected to biofeedback instruments.

After I lead groups in a mind-body exploration on only one side of the body, people often beg me to balance them by anchoring them in the opposing side, as well. As I look at the audience, I often see many participants now have one shoulder remarkably lower than their other shoulder. They are leaning to one side as well! Many people are astonished that their minds have that much impact. Because being this present in only half of the body can be very annoying, I quickly lead them through progressive muscle relaxation on the opposite side to help balance them.

In the first mind-body exploration of this book, I will invite you to make a similar comparison in your body. You will find that in these more profound states of consciousness, you will become aware of things within yourself that you didn't even know were happening. Such realizations are crucial to our process: throughout this book, I will be encouraging you to come to know your internal energetic landscape, and giving you methods for enhancing it. There is a world of activity occurring underneath your nose. I will be teaching you the skills to engage with it powerfully.

You will also learn that this work is simple but not easy. It seems simple to hold your mind in the body until, very quickly, it is not! Most of us suffer from a horrible monkey mind, our minds jumping from topic to topic as we subconsciously drag our bodies along. This work reveals our lack of mental discipline. We learn that our mind-body habits are not only not serving us but are severely sabotaging us, as well. Until we can stay in command of our mind, we have little chance of staying in control of our lives and even less control over our happiness levels.

Fascinatingly, as people practice this work, their courage simultaneously expands exponentially due to the greater mental discipline, inward presence, and self-respect it fosters. One client, who was practicing these mind-body explorations between three biofeedback appointments, demonstrated the unwavering confidence and self-efficacy this work engenders. Asked how she was doing with her new biofeedback skills, she quipped, "I am doing great. I have lowered my blood pressure, reduced my need for insulin, and I can sleep at night without sleeping pills. Now I want to know what else can I do?"

This empowered state of well-being precisely demonstrates what happens as people learn to come into masterful command of their nervous system. Coming into control of their bodies' physiology, they come into control of themselves. Their improved mental focus and clarity allow people to direct their efforts more strategically, so they have more resources to be effective. This focal shift is similar to the difference between cutting tissue with a light bulb versus a laser. They are both lights, but one is focused light, strong enough to make an incision. This book will teach you how to focus your mind so it becomes strong enough, similar to a laser, to make effective changes. Before proceeding to the next chapter, please perform the one-sided mind-body exploration five times so that you can experience the powerful impact of your focused mind.

You can find the mind-body exploration audio downloads here: ConsciousnessAthletes.com.

Enter the password: explore

At the end of each chapter, I will offer practical tools for transferring and integrating what you are learning in the Consciousness Athlete curriculum into daily life. Please see notes for this chapter on the next page.

Chapter One Notes:
Conditioning Your Body For Happiness
By Transferring Consciousness Athlete Skills
into Daily Life

Please listen to the mind-body exploration, Skillfully Altering Inner Space, for this chapter 5 times.

Be sure to grasp the difference between thoroughly maintaining awareness in your body versus vacating it.

We feel happiness in our bodies, not our minds.

Through the Consciousness Athlete process, we are in a version of athletic training to condition our body's nervous system for sustaining heightened states of well-being.

As we face stressful situations in our lives, we are unaware of how much we tighten and contract our bodies.

The quickest way to stop the stress response is to become aware of your body in space as you make efforts to release tension.

Begin practicing maintaining an awareness of your body during typical daily activities, especially if you are stressed.

For instance, feel your feet as you are walking down the hallway, or become aware of the surface under your legs and behind your back when you are sitting on a chair

When under stress, immediately become aware of your breathing.

Are you breathing? Probably not.

Our instinctive stress response is often to stop breathing, especially when we are paying bills. Notice your breathing pattern the next time you pull out your checkbook or pay your bills online.

If your stress response causes you to breathe too fast, be sure to slow your breathing down before it escalates into full-blown anxiety.

Essentially, anxiety is a body phenomenon, not a mental one.

When we take command of our nervous system, we learn to lead the body into states completely incompatible with anxiety, which makes it virtually impossible for fear to grow into overwhelm.

Be sure to practice these essential skills before proceeding to the next chapter. If you don't, you will not have the basic mastery skills established in your nervous system to accomplish the more advanced techniques as we progress.

Also, remember - Have fun exploring your new orientation to life!

It is only the beginning of good things!

Please visit consciousnessathletes.com/explorations

Enter the password: explore

CHAPTER 2 - OK, SO WHERE DO I ANCHOR MY MIND IN MY BODY?

Ideally, you will be reading this chapter after practicing the "one-sided" body-mind audio exploration. You would have experienced the distinct difference of anchoring your consciousness inside the body versus having it run without boundaries. When your mind anchors in the body, you are present. There is a lot of talk in self-help groups about being present, and often people don't quite understand what it means to be "in the now." To state it succinctly, being present means that your mind is where your body is. Research has demonstrated that when our consciousness is "present," we are generally happier.

But first, let's talk about why becoming present is so much easier said than done! As we discuss this, let's also take any shame out of our struggle with being present. Some people may find it very easy, but most others struggle. Well-intentioned people sometimes chide those they see suffering, telling them to "just let it go" or "be here now," but without really understanding the intricate skill of being present. This unskilled criticism can leave people feeling unheard, judged, or too embarrassed to share their feelings.

Because humans have a higher capacity than animals to think and create, it is often more difficult for us to maintain present awareness. Our neocortex keeps us busy performing complex functions, such as conscious thought and language. These mental activities entertain our attention during daily tasks. Instead of being present to our mundane tasks, our mind often wanders. As we grocery shop, we may worry about a family situation or be reliving unresolved issues of the workday on our commute home.

Research scientists have learned that when our mind is not focused on a task, it often wanders to not very good places! A Harvard study interviewed 2,250 subjects ranging in ages from 18 to 88, representing a wide range of socioeconomic backgrounds and occupations, to determine how engaged their minds were with their current task. The researchers learned that almost half of the time, the current activity did not fully involve the subject's thoughts. Researchers checked in with subjects at random times via a phone app and recorded what they were doing at that moment and on what their mind was focused. They determined that the test subjects often had wandering minds: almost 47% of the time! For instance, if the study participants were grocery shopping, they could not think about their shopping list. They were often ruminating about their work, families, or other topics.

Moreover, the same study reported that not being present in the moment was the cause of reported unhappiness, not the consequence. One of the researchers, Matthew Killingsworth, noted: "Mind-wandering is an excellent predictor of people's happiness. In fact, how often our minds leave the present is a better predictor of our happiness than the activities in which we're engaged."

Mind-wandering causes unhappiness because our minds rarely meander into pleasant places! Our nervous system has a negativity bias, also known as the negativity effect. This effect describes the hard-wired impulse within all of us that, even when of equal intensity, things of a more negative nature have a more significant effect on our psychological state and processes than neutral or positive things. This hard-wired propensity to dwell on negativity is why we often leave work and forget all of the positive inter-actions during the day, while our mind wanders into reviewing one brief, negative situation.

When our minds are not focused on a task, the part of the brain that becomes activated as we rumi-nate is called the default mode network (DMN). Analyzing tour thoughts' quality when our mind wanders, researchers have categorized them into four general categories of thinking which will probably sound very familiar to you as I list them here. When our minds meander, we often 1) rehash unresolved conflicts of our past, 2) agonize about the future, 3) worry how we appear to others, and 4) narrate, or often, criticize our lives. Do those topics sound familiar to you? When I present this information to audiences, I see a lot of heads nodding. It is important to note that the DMN can also be utilized for positive results. Because of the DMN's ability to review and analyze, it can be an excellent problem-solving tool. If the DMN is left unattended, however, it runs us amok at breakneck speeds, spinning out its constant internal chatter—often referred to as the "inner critic," or what I refer to as the "inner terrorist."

There is an opposing network to the DMN in the brain, referred to as the task-positive network (TPN). Our TPN gets activated when we focus on a task, which often silences the cranky, meandering DMN. When we take charge of the locus of our awareness and activate the TPN, it can be remarkable how swiftly our mood shifts.

I often teach in schools with under-served children. Since many of them struggle with focus, I strive relentlessly, often against their open resistance, to harness their focus. I am passionate about reigning in their attention because I know that when teaching them how to focus, I am teaching them how to be happy. A focused mind is generally a happy mind. Each week I look for ways to inspire them to want to bring their thoughts into greater focus. Because I am so committed and not easily discouraged, I usually succeed in helping them move toward greater inner peace and self-awareness. To help them become more familiar and adept at navigating internal space, I ask them to compare how they felt before and after the focusing exercise. The students often report how amazed they are at their improvement of mood.

Ancient teachers were well aware of this phenomenon—that focus enhances mood and well-being—which is why the technology of meditation has survived millennia. Centuries ago, people did not have lights, television, cell phones, or the internet to occupy their minds when the sun went down. There was not much to entertain them during the night except sit in the dark and think. Without external entertainment, they often studied the internal meanderings of their minds. Instead of allowing their DMN's nagging voice to run rampant with fear and worry, they discovered ways to conquer negative proclivities by focusing their thoughts and activating the TPN. This was the beginning of the world's ancient meditation traditions.

In the mind-body audio exploration for this chapter, we will practice activating the task-positive network by focusing our mind on the body. This internal focus discourages the DMN's tendency to run amok. We will stop the mind's blathering by activating the TPN through becoming focused. We will also learn to focus our awareness at various strategic places in the body to alter our state of being dramatically. When we change where our mind is anchored in the body, we change our entire orientation to life. You will be delighted to learn that you have far more power over how you feel that you have ever been taught.

The first place in the body where we will anchor our minds is in the lower abdomen, which martial artists consider the seat of power within us. As we cultivate this area with awareness, we gain an impressive equanimity and strength. For centuries, eastern warriors cultivated understanding of their power center to maintain balance and focus during war. When martial artists perform amazing feats, such as breaking boards with their feet or making their bodies so heavy their opponents can't move them. They accomplish these feats by becoming hyper-focused on their power center. In Japan, this center is referred to as the hara, and in China, it is called the tan tien. The tan tien is located in the lower abdomen, about 1.5 inches below your belly button. This area is also the center of gravity of the body.

When we anchor our mind in the lower abdomen,

we are accessing more than just a physical center. We are accessing an electrical power center of the body's acupuncture meridians as well. Acupuncture is an ancient Chinese medicine-based approach that has proven to help various health conditions by triggering specific points on the body with needles. These points are on meridian lines, which are invisible energetic pathways, or channels, that run through the body. For centuries medical philosophies have espoused that "qi"(chi) or vital life force runs through these meridians, and anything that disrupts the smooth flow of qi is said to cause illness. Meridians are often stimulated to increase life force distribution with needles. However, it is interesting to note that we can also stimulate these meridians with our minds

When we anchor our minds in the lower abdomen, we are "stirring the pot," so to speak, of our vital life force, which causes a healthy mental fertile stillness. The ancient Taoists referred to this area as the gate of life. They considered it the most crucial gateway for physical health and strength because all major acupuncture meridians travel through this point in the body. Mantak Chia, one of the world's leading authorities on the body's subtle energies, refers to the tan tien as the "fundamental power storehouse of the body." It is a center of potential. When you learn how to tap into your tan tien with your mind, you feel it is a dynamic activity center. Subjectively, when you finally can park your awareness there, it may feel comforting, like "home."

In Eastern medicine, the tan tien is considered to be a battery, elixir, and pump. It is referred to as a battery because it holds a charge of chi or life force. This philosophy assumes that we are all born with an amount of individual "natal chi" or energy stored in the tan tien. The tan tien is considered an elixir because it mixes the three significant types of subtle energies that pass through our bodies. Chinese medical theory refers to these as chi, jing, and shen and refers to these different energies as the three treasures because they are considered responsible for our lives' quality. If we have an imbalance of these energies, we feel imbalanced. The tan tien is also considered to be a pump because it pumps this elixir out to the rest of the body to nourish us.

When we focus our awareness in the tan tien, we are physically balanced in the body, which interestingly means that we are far more emotionally balanced as well. Our intention is crisp, clear, and unfettered, without entanglements. In fact, the tan tien is often considered the "seat of intention." There is much discussion about intention in our culture recently, but the mysteries of intention have long been explored in the East. Eastern health and martial arts practitioners strive to maintain an awareness of their tan tien as much as possible. This understanding is so culturally ingrained that if a Japanese boy throws a temper tantrum, his mother may scold him by saying "Hara. Hara!" meaning "Belly. Belly!" The Japanese mother would be encouraging her child to get focused and become present and calm by anchoring his mind in his abdomen.

Psychologist Karlfried Graf Durkheim spent the years between 1938-1947 studying Japanese culture and observed the reliance on the hara in everyday life. In his book, Hara, the Vital Centre of Man, Durkheim describes the "matured inwardness" of individuals who have spent years harnessing their mind's awareness to their hara. Life simply does not rattle these individuals. When anchored in the tan tien, they remain as calm as deep ocean waters, even if they can hear the noise of violent waves. Durkheim also writes that people who have a robust hara presence have a powerful influence over others. Often, people with strong hara are very sexy! They are charismatic and have a magnanimousness about them, which draws people to them. Martin Luther King is an example of someone who was anchored in his hara, as evidenced by his relentless commitment to making his dream a reality, especially during challenging times. Gandhi had great hara as well. These leaders had a steadfast commitment to social change, and influenced others through their unwavering intention. This invincible dedication is a natural outgrowth of being firmly grounded in the hara. However, it is important to note that just because people have a healthy hara, it does not mean they have purified their intentions. It only means that they are more effective in achieving their purposes. People like cult leader David Koresh had a strong hara as well! Every now and then, I see someone swagger with the confidence that only comes from being deeply anchored in the hara. Recognizing that state of being does not mean to automatically trust them. They are still enjoyable to watch!

I teach people how to tether their minds' awareness in their hara by having them stand on two rubber discs that can be found in most public gyms. When they establish their balance on these discs, they can become aware of their tan tien in their lower abdomen. Through this exercise, the tan tien becomes a tangible place in the body, not just a theoretical construct. After they become balanced on the discs by anchoring their awareness to their tan tiens, I strategically ask them to tell me about the most stressful issues they are facing. As they start to answer me, they become imbalanced and wobble, often falling off the discs with laughter. Clients struggle to get back on the discs and remain upright while we pursue the topic further. It is such a clear demonstration that when they are physically balanced, they are emotionally balanced. They become aware of what anchoring in the hara means when they lose their balance while mentally confronting a particular situation. You could also say that they lose their power, as they become physically weakened while reviewing their stressors.

There is a way to maintain our power while thinking about challenging topics. As clients learn how to stay in their tan tien while reviewing stressful issues, the quality of their thinking changes, to a surprising degree. It is fascinating to listen to what clients say about stressful topics as they learn to remain anchored in their tan tien. Their thoughts pivot from victimized thinking to creative thinking. People become detached from their struggles. Their perspectives change to become more philosophical and transcendent. This integrated and innovative thinking is the signature that they are thinking from a balanced tan tien.

An example of individuals not anchored in their tan tien would be those who struggle with substance abuse. Because the addiction struggle often causes people to disassociate from their bodies, addicts do not have a firm awareness of their tan tien. Their minds are easily plucked by external stimuli, including trigger foods or addictive substances, so it is difficult for them to gather their awareness back in their body. In fact, clients who exhibit substance abuse often fall off the bubble discs when they talk about their addictive substance of choice. I even had to catch a woman as she fell off the discs and on to the ground after thinking about her passion for chocolate chip cookies! This loss of physical stability demonstrates to them that they lose their balance, both physically and mentally, in the presence of their substance of choice. They become acutely aware of how they surrender their power, unable to maintain their center in its presence. I have witnessed the same phenomenon with the Galvanic Skin Response (GSR) instrument. The GSR pitch often starts to squeal if people talk about their trigger substances while connected to the instrument.

The goal of our work together will be to develop the internal mental control to maintain a general awareness of our tan tien, especially during the difficult moments of our lives. We can think of cultivating this awareness as being rooted or tethered to our tan tien, our center of gravity of our bodies with the earth. By remaining anchored in our lower abdomen, we have the strength of will to maintain equanimity, even when life is severely challenging us. Learning to tether our minds to the tan tien during stress, we appreciate having a safe place to land mentally and emotionally, as we consider appropriate, more resourceful responses. Consider how large trees remain stable through the storms of many seasons. The tree can only grow big and tall because it has a broad, rich root structure underneath. The roots of large trees ground them so well they do not bend or fall even in the harshest of winds. To maintain our power in the body, we must gain roots in our tan tien. Our focus on the tan tien as the center of gravity in the body, tethers us to the earth in a similar manner. In the exploration for this chapter, we will be working toward establishing a firm awareness of the tan tien, enabling us to remain resolute in the face of chaos as a tree stands tall during hazardous storms.

I am passionate about teaching these internal skills of remaining anchored in the body because I have witnessed how learning this skill changes people's lives trajectories. I am saddened that I have not seen these skills taught anywhere within this context, which is why people often tragically struggle unnecessarily for decades. It brings me great pleasure to teach children these skills. I hope that they will not need to spend years fighting against themselves as I witness many adults. I love to teach children in schools this esoteric skill of anchoring in their hara by having them face common real-life challenges. I often bring candy with me, as an opportunity for students to tether their minds in their tan tien in the face of temptation. I purposely buy three bags—one for each type of sweet tooth—sweet, sour, and chocolate! If you have guessed that my approach to mindfulness is a little unorthodox, you are right! I don't linger on basic mindfulness practices too long before integrating more significant and meaningful biofeedback and character-building themes by applying self-mastery skills to gritty real-life challenges. I do this because we learn the most when we are grappling with our most intimidating struggles. We may think we have control of our minds, but challenges reveal areas of our mind's weaknesses. Biofeedback instruments show our raw responses to challenges and astonishingly demonstrate that the body does not lie.

I pass out three small pieces of candy per child, with the instruction that if they can hold back from the temptation to eat the candy, I will give them three more small pieces 15 minutes later. In the interim, we discuss what is happening in their bodies as they are tempted to eat the candy. I remember one fourth-grader lamenting, in a comical voice, that she was "suffering" as she resisted the urge not to eat the candy in front of her. Her antics were funny at first. However, she continued after the humor had worn off. I reminded her that the student next to her was not suffering, because he was looking away from the candy, and neither was the child on the other side of her, who had hidden the candy under a piece of paper to avoid temptation. She was "suffering" because she had allowed her mind to anchor in her suffering. As students struggle with temptation, I ask them to anchor their minds in their tan tien. Simultaneously, I encourage them to allow their rapidly growing self-respect to emerge into their awareness. I see their backs straighten as they feel the pride of mental discipline. I love these moments!

In the mind-body audio exploration created to accompany this chapter, Poise and Power, I will teach you how to hold a stance toward life grounded in your tan tien. As you review complex relationships, situations, and addictions, you will learn how to maintain your awareness steady in your tan tien, and observe the powerful change in your consciousness. Practicing this place of being, you will become "awed" by what it truly means to be "empowered." While you cultivate this mastery, you will often feel a profound wave of self-respect and satisfaction move into your consciousness. You may even encounter a state of being that you have never experienced before. Still, you will immediately realize that it feels familiar, and that you like it.

We are beginning to cultivate the discipline of mind required to influence our nervous system significantly. We gain greater mastery and control through this discipline, as we intentionally create a calmer internal environment. This philosophical perspective enables us to consider a broader range of responsive behaviors, facilitating feelings of embodied empowerment.

Before we anchor in the tan tien, we will begin by

aligning with the body's vertical power current of energy, by sitting as upright as possible. To become aware of our tan tien, we want to feel balanced in the body from front to back, and from left to right. We will also begin by aligning with an imaginary plumb line, starting about 1.5 feet above our head and ending between our legs, below our feet, with a weight at the end. We will practice holding our heads high and shoulders back with great dignity. As the founder of Shambala Meditation, Chogyam Trungpa Rinpoche taught, we will sit with "good head and shoulders." I have done this with students in school as well. I invite them to sit with their legs crisscrossed on the floor. With their permission, I run my thumb up their spine between their shoulder blades. Their shoulders splay back and down, and more than once, the room of students quietly gasp at the majestic beauty and dignity that naturally springs forth from the model student. We are all touched by this experience.

When we are fully present, we naturally hold our head and shoulders with this regal air. The research of psychology professor, Richard Petty, reveals that when we hold our head up, we have an easier time thinking "empowering, positive" thoughts about ourselves. Conversely, when we have our heads down, we are more likely to experience "hopeless, helpless, powerless, and negative" feelings about ourselves. Petty surmises that the marked increase of time spent sitting in front of computers and looking down at smartphones may be a significant contributing factor to the rise of depression in recent years. Because vision is lowered and eyes gaze down so much, it is easy to become self-centered. Our mood may also be negatively altered when we slump because when our head droops, our chest collapses, severely restricting our breathing. This lack of oxygenation in the body can lead to lethargy and depression as well. I invite students to walk with confidence, with their heads up, as if they know where they are going in life. When we lift our heads and see others, we take attention off ourselves. We naturally create an open heart, which is the subject of our next chapter.

Enjoy this next mind-body exploration, *Poise and Power*, because it will reconnect you to your inherent dignity and worth. But don't just practice experiencing your inherent dignity during the *Poise and Power* exploration. Continue exploring the possibilities of this new orientation to the world as you walk into work, have difficult conversations with your spouse, or coaxing your resistant teenager. Explore these profound states of being and how they offer you a more extensive, more empowering range of responses. Feel appreciation for yourself and gain a tremendous respect for your choices. When people try to rattle you, make it a game to see how much you can remain anchored in your tan tien while breathing deep into the belly, like a bellows. In the face of a tempting food or drink, practice keeping your awareness rooted in the tan tien, and do not allow your consciousness to hemorrhage toward the temptation.

There will still be difficult days when it is incredibly challenging to maintain focus. But every time you attempt maintaining an awareness of your tan tien, whether you feel you have been successful or not, you will have gained an enormous step toward mastery. Some people may not be up for this challenge, and that is understandable. It will require grit and will. It requires that you take a stand for yourself and your happiness. It requires you to honor yourself and consider yourself worthy of relentlessly pursuing your own well-being. As I often say, this type of grace does not come cheap. If you just read this book and don't practice the internal skills, you will not make many strides. However, I guarantee that if you take a stand internally to maintain your physical and emotional center, your self-respect will grow immensely. I urge you to honor yourself in this way. It is only the beginning of a more empowering orientation to life.

I guarantee that if you practice the skill of silencing the unhealthy mind-wandering of the default mode network by activating the task-positive network through keeping your awareness focused in your abdomen, your confidence will bloom. You will gain much greater mastery of your mind, and it will show in your increased self-respect. Your decision-making will improve without having to white-knuckle healthier choices. You will want to do the right thing because it feels like the right thing, within the deepest part of your being, and you will be unwilling to turn against yourself. You will become addicted to feeling aligned and no longer be willing to give up this feeling of inherent honor for anything. You can find the audio download *Poise and Power* at ConsciousnessAthletes.com.

Enter the password: explore

Chapter Two Notes:
Conditioning Your Body For Happiness
By Transferring Consciousness Athlete Skills
into Daily Life

Please listen to the mind-body exploration, *Poise and Power*, for this chapter 5 times

Practice anchoring your mind deep in your abdomen, approximately 1.5 inches below your navel, as you review difficult challenges in your life.

I strongly suggest purchasing balance discs to hone this skill.

Put one foot on each disc about 1.5 feet apart.

Slightly bend your knees to help establish your balance.

Now bring to mind any stressful situation in your life, and practice maintaining your physical balance.

When you start to wobble, bring your awareness to your legs and lower abdomen.

You may need to unearth some mental grit to maintain your center.

Don't just give up. Stay with it until you can hold your center.

As you remain anchored in your lower abdomen, notice how your thinking evolves.

You may start to feel more detached from the situation.

As you distance yourself from the difficult

emotions, notice if you find yourself becoming more resourceful.

Because you have created more generous space within your consciousness, you will have more mental bandwidth for creative solutions to emerge.

If you are unable to purchase balance discs,

simply sit and place your hand on your lower abdomen.

1.5 inches below your navel.

Feel the heat of your hand on the area of the tan tien.

Practice tethering your awareness there.

Now bring to mind any stressor while being sure to maintain your locus of awareness in your lower abdomen.

If your awareness frequently pops out of your tan tien space,

continue leading it back until you can think about the stressor

without your mind flickering.

Finally, if you are tempted by food, drink, drugs, or behaviors, be sure to hold your awareness in the lower abdomen in the presence of temptation.

Feel what it is like to hold your power and allow any feelings of dignity and self-respect to emerge.

Please   visit consciousnessathletes.com/explorations

Enter the password: explore

CHAPTER 3 - HEART HYGIENE
FOR FACILITATING
EMOTIONAL FREEDOM

Life can be challenging. Have you noticed it?

As we move through the life cycle, we have multiple experiences of love and loss, trust and betrayal, ambition, and surrender. We have to learn how to live and work with people very different from us. We struggle to understand how to meet our own needs while striving to meet the needs of others. Throughout the trials and tribulations, we learn how words have a profound impact to hurt or heal. The residue of all these troubling experiences creates what I refer to as "scar tissue on our hearts." I mean that both physically and emotionally. In this chapter, we will learn powerful tools to remove scar tissue on our hearts so we can feel the innocence of children again, no matter what calamities we endured in the past. We will return to this innocence by learning how to liberate our hearts. For instance, take a moment right now and think about someone who you feel has betrayed you. Take a moment and remember the nuances of the situation. Notice how your entire interior changed when you recalled this situation. I know it may feel uncomfortable, but if you can gather a little bit of courage to do it, you will gain powerful information. Where do you feel yourself clutching in the body? For many of you, the area in your body that is contracting is within or near your heart center.

Most of us have no idea how much clutching in the heart center casts a very dark cloud over our mood. Maybe you just noticed it. You were reading along in the book and probably feeling okay or a sense of well-being. Then, I asked you to pull up a negative memory, and a storm of emotion may have taken over you. To stop that storm of emotion from overwhelming you, you may have tightened or clutched in the body, often in the heart. Clutching the heart almost seems like a primal instinct at times. However, as we will learn, when we smother negative feelings in the heart, we repress our joy as well.

Do you remember how we discussed that we feel feelings in our bodies, not our minds? Understand that emotions of suffering are not just a thought process. They are a body phenomenon as well, especially in our hearts. Emotional pain even alters the quality of our physical heart rate. Negative emotion causes our hearts to beat with low heart rate variability, which researchers have determined is associated with psychological impediments, such as anxiety, depression, and post-traumatic stress disorders. Our heart rate influences mood because the heart is the strongest oscillating signal in the body. The heart emits the most powerful electromagnetic signal in the body, one that is so strong; it can be measured on your toes...and beyond! When we change the quality of our heart's beat-to-beat changes, we influence our entire body and, thus, our mood.

Take a moment to digest how empowering this information can be because it reveals the converse is true. When we improve our heart rate variability, we release our suffering and feel more joy. How cool is that? We learn we don't have to feel persecuted by our life's circumstances if we take control of our nervous system. By consciously manipulating our heart rate variability, we lead our entire body and mind into a more harmonious state, without years of therapy!

For almost thirty years, the Institute of Heartmath has performed dozens of research studies demonstrating how negative emotions, such as stress, anger, and frustration, negatively influence our heart rate variability. They have also shown that positive emotions, such as appreciation, love, and care, enhance heart health. Heartmath's data has been exciting because it demonstrates that when we take conscious control of our heart rate variability, meaning beat-to-beat changes in heart rate, we take command of our moods.

A study in the American Journal of Cardiology demonstrated when stressed workers learned how to control their heart rate variability, they were able to not only significantly lower their blood pressure but also improved their emotional health. These workers experienced a 25% improvement in their ability to focus, a 45% reduction in exhaustion, and a 41% reduction in their intention to leave the job. Take a moment and pause to think about the implications of this study. By merely anchoring our minds' awareness in our hearts in a skilled manner, we enhance our focus, become less tired, and experience greater peace in the present moment. We gain all of these benefits without paying a cent or taking medication with harmful side effects. When I think about all these benefits, I always find myself saying, "Sign me up!"

Increasing heart rate variability is amazingly simple. We will continue to anchor our mind in the body as we have been learning. However, in this chapter, we will learn how to anchor awareness in our energetic heart, located in the center of our chest. While holding attention in our chest, we will synch our breathing with our heart rate by inhaling and exhaling in equally measured breaths. For instance, we breathe in for five counts and breathe out for five counts while maintaining awareness in our chest. According to Heartmath's research, after we establish this synchronization, the next step is to invoke restorative emotions such as appreciation, love, or care. These positive emotions restore us back to remembering our wholeness. Through this simple process, we stabilize our emotional state. We come into greater command of our moods as we learn to reliably shift into more harmonious states on demand.

One reason why heart rhythms influence mood so much is that our heart emits the body's most powerful oscillating signal. Our hearts' signal is so strong it is calculated not only from everywhere on the body but also from a few feet away from the body. Amazingly, Heartmath documented that our heart rate may be measured influencing the people's brainwaves. When we observe one person's brain waves, we may pick up the heartbeat of another person nearby. So, how we manage our hearts influences our moods and could also affect the attitudes of those people around us.

Healthy heart rate variability means that the time between heartbeats is erratic or highly variable in healthy hearts. If this phenomenon seems counterintuitive, you did hear me correctly. If the time between our heartbeats is consistent, we are more prone to depression and heart disease. In daily life, when we experience the stress response, our hearts are unable to be flexible with our environment, which causes extra wear and tear on our hearts.

The heart's signal is so powerful that it even influences our emotional flexibility, as well. The field of neurocardiology is documenting how our hearts do not merely circulate blood; they also contribute to our mood. Like the rest of our nervous system, the heart has 40,000 nerve cells that scan our environments for new possibilities and understandings. When we experience higher heart rate variability, the heart's highly charged electrical activity makes it a sensitive instrument that searches for fresh opportunities to respond to our environments in meaningful and creative interactions with those around us.

We have all experienced emotional trauma at some point in our lives. When we experience distress, our heart rate variability decreases, meaning that our hearts are no longer flexible in their ability to respond to their environment. Duke Researcher Simon Beacon performed groundbreaking work documenting this phenomenon in coronary artery disease patients. He writes, "We found that during times of mental stress and negative emotions, the participants' hearts showed a reduced capacity to respond." Essentially, stress puts our hearts in lockdown, causing the time between the heart's beats to become more rigid and consistent. Beacon writes, "Sick hearts show very little heart rate variability, so they are not as responsive, leaving them vulnerable. Healthy hearts have a better ability to respond to anything that occurs. The bottom line is that the unmanaged stress we experience throughout the day can be bad for our hearts." Reduced heart rate variability is a sign of disease, both physical and psychological. Patients who suffer from depression and post-traumatic stress disorder have very low heart rate variability. Researchers surmise heart rate variability is a plausible mechanism to explain why depression is such a strong risk factor for heart disease.

As we progress in life, it is easy to acquire emotional scar tissue on our hearts. We experience life's inevitable betrayals, from children, spouses, family, co-workers, employment, and even our bodies. You simply can't breathe and be immune from the dark side of being human. Our heart rate variability can be a mirror that reveals how well we manage the endless challenges and losses we face. The Institute of Heartmath's research suggests that heart rate variability significantly decreases if we acquire lots of unresolved emotional issues over our lifetime. If we accumulate excessive hard feelings toward others, we reduce our heart rate variability at an accelerated rate. Simon's study found that even small fluctuations in heart rate variability can have a negative cumulative impact.

One of the primary skills of becoming a Consciousness Athlete is cultivating the ability to maintain what I refer to as "heart hygiene," which I consider to be the systematic, intentional release of our hearts from the stranglehold of unprocessed negative emotion. It is essential to understand that managing our hearts is very similar to maintaining a garden. If a garden is not weeded regularly, the weeds will strangle the vegetables. If a garden is not watered regularly, the plants will not grow. If there is not enough sunshine, plants will not grow nearly to their full potential. Our hearts are incredibly similar. If we don't weed our hearts of resentments and hurt, our hearts are incapable of feeling our maximum capacity for joy. If we don't water our hearts with good people and wholesome information, our hearts will not have the nourishment to grow. If we don't expose our hearts to the equivalent of emotional sunshine, our hearts will not grow toward an orientation of light and love. I can't stress this enough: the repercussions of ignoring the needs of our hearts are enormous.

However, in this chapter, I will offer you the best tool I know to cleanse and uplift the heart. We will eliminate the excessive accumulation of scar tissue on our hearts by adapting tools that I refer to as part of a "dynamic lifestyle of forgiveness." I consider this to be a "forgiveness technology" that is highly effective. Many of us were raised in homes where we were taught through our spiritual training that we must forgive, but we were never instructed how to forgive. Unfortunately, many of us interpreted our childhood lessons of forgiveness such that we were supposed to repress negative emotions and pretend that the bad situations never happened. Those traumas did happen, and our heart's cell tissue keeps the score. However, with this forgiveness tool, you can renew your heart in a manner that will liberate you from this ancient oppression. This will help you sustain your emotional freedom through all of your future challenges as well.

This work is immediate and highly effective, but it is not a form of spiritual bypassing because it is a skill that moves awareness down into the body, where the resentment is embedded. In other words, it removes hurt from its root. We will move attention into our hearts to skillfully experience and release negative emotions. This emotional release will allow us to feel lighthearted again! You see, good feelings are always available. It is our negativity that keeps them at bay. Think of good feelings as being present in your body, but they are like an underwater buoy. When the resistance on the float lifts, the buoy shoots up out of the water. There is a similar process that occurs in the heart. When we release binding negative emotions, well-being inevitably surges to the surface as if it has been waiting for us to release it all along!

This work has been so powerful that I now make sure I never go more than 24 hours without doing some type of forgiveness or release work. I consider this work to be as important as taking a daily shower. It gives a similar clean feeling to my spirit as well! I am dedicated to this discipline because I find that my mood baseline continues to increase. I simply don't feel the low moods I experienced as a young woman. When I actively do heart work, I feel buoyant and find myself smiling for no good reason. When we set an intention to move toward having the heart rate variability, or open heart of a child, our mood immediately responds. I believe that this is what Jesus was referring to when he spoke about how children are closer to experiencing the kingdom of God within. In the gospel of Luke, Jesus says, "Allow the little children to come to me, and don't hinder them, for the Kingdom of God belongs to such as these. Most certainly, I tell you, whoever doesn't receive the Kingdom of God like a little child, he will in no way enter into it."

There is no doubt, an open heart, a truly open heart, generates sweet nectar in the body, and I have personally witnessed how children live with more of this nectar, even if it doesn't appear they show it. Researchers have determined that children have considerably higher heart rate variability than adults. We can witness this when we observe children's ability to laugh and enjoy everyday experiences more, even after trauma. With their high heart rate variability, children are much closer to experiencing elevated emotions. I have even witnessed some of the most dysregulated kids have higher heart rate variability than their teachers and counselors. Unfortunately, HRV naturally decreases over our life span. After experiencing the dark side of human nature over the decades our hearts often close up, like daylilies at the end of the day, when darkness comes. If we leave our hearts unattended, we can sentence ourselves to a life of what Henry David Thoreau referred to as quiet desperation. This is because the heart is also where we experience hurt as well as joy, so the tender beauty of an open heart becomes obscured due to its fragile nature.

Although the research reveals that heart rate variability decreases with age, it is possible to renew our innocence again by cultivating a dynamic lifestyle of freedom through daily forgiveness and release. This lifestyle did not come easily for me. Before I could reap its endless benefits, I needed to understand the technical aspects of forgiveness. I went on a relentless pursuit to regain my buoyant heart because of my deep desire to reconcile disappointments of betrayal. I was unwilling to resign to having a governor on my good feelings due to past disappointments. Such a life of muted contentment was entirely unacceptable to me, and I hope it is for you as well. My deep knowledge and understanding of the mind-body phenomenon enabled me to make such a resolute decision. I am highly skilled at navigating inner space, and I was entirely confident this was possible for me. I intend that by the time you finish this book, you gain the same confidence in your ability to foster good feelings. I hope to accelerate your emotional liberation by sharing the technology of forgiveness with you in this chapter. If you feel emotionally stuck, the mind-body exploration for this chapter will help you move through stale feelings, so you can create again from the vibrancy and zest of a child's unrestrained heart.

The first strategy of forgiveness is to recognize its benefits. Research has shown that forgiveness enhances our health in at least two ways. One is by reducing nasty stress hormones generated when we feel hostility, fear, or resentment. Stress also puts our health in danger by increasing the risks of hypertension, heart attack, and stroke. When we feel resentment, our bodies release a cascade of stress hormones that narrow focus, decrease problem-solving abilities, and just generally make us feel like victims. Stress increases our pain levels. It has been determined that forgiveness can even reduce back pain. Researchers found that those who have chronic back pain and who have chosen to forgive others experience lower levels of pain, anger, and depression than those who have not forgiven. When we genuinely forgive, we enjoy healthier relationships and dramatically enhance our health and happiness. "In a way," cardiologist Dr. Ornish says, "the most selfish thing you can do for yourself is to forgive other people."

The research team led by Due Zheng of Erasmus Univesity's Rotterdam School of Management demonstrated that forgiveness makes us happier and makes us physically stronger. Researchers found that participants could jump higher in an ostensible fitness test after people performed a forgiveness exercise than when people were primed to feel resentment. These findings suggest unforgiveness causes an actual workload for the body that forgiveness releases. This research provides evidence that forgiveness can help victims overcome the adverse effects of conflict.

I hope I am inspiring you to want to let go of old stories of loss and betrayal, to release the good feelings inside of you. If you still are not convinced you want to forgive, I have more reasons for why you may want to consider it. What if I told you there was objective evidence that forgiveness made you happier? Would you want to pursue it more? I hope so!

When we increase heart rate variability, our brains change to emit more alpha brain waves associated with high creativity, compassion, insight, love, happiness, and general well-being. 40 Years of Zen is a powerful electroencephalographic (EEG) training protocol that focuses almost exclusively on the power of forgiveness to lift happiness levels through extensive brainwave training. They claim that using their forgiveness methods, brain waves of participants shift to patterns of someone who has spent 21 to 40 years of practicing Zen meditation. The 40 Years of Zen practice fosters a heightened focus by increasing those desirable alpha waves in the brain. The designers of the program discovered that the single most significant factor suppressing alpha waves is holding on to grudges and anger. Participants, who pay the $15,000 fee, learn to increase their alpha waves by focusing on one thing...you guessed it...forgiveness!

Attendees are encouraged to forgive every person who they ever felt wronged them—even if it was only in the slightest way imaginable—including parents, former teachers, or even waiters whose name they never knew! Vishen Lakhiani, the founder of Mind-Valley.com, completed the program and reported that his alpha waves would spike every time he did a round of forgiveness. Because he saw such a dramatic benefit, he strived to release every last bit of resentment out of his system to gain higher alpha brainwave amplitudes.

Forgiveness may seem a formidable task, but not if

we consider it strictly from the body's perspective. I know I have forgiven someone if I can think of someone and not have my body contract when I think of him or her. To be clear, I still have the memory, but I don't have the sucker punch feeling in my body. In the mind-body exploration of this chapter, we will release bodily constrictions of the energetic heart, which improves heart rate variability to enhance our ability to forgive.

The reduced HRV of unforgiveness gives great credence to the phrase "resentment is like swallowing poison and expecting the other person to die." As we start living the dynamic lifestyle of forgiveness, we can no longer tolerate carrying grudges. We learn to savor and appreciate the buoyant feelings of a liberated heart. Why would we give those good feelings up for anyone? Especially for the people who have already burdened us? It becomes evident through pure logic that resentments do not serve us in the long term after we have processed the wisdom of the situation. As we see this clearly, we become far less willing to hold any resentment.

I understand if you find forgiveness daunting. Humans sometimes perform heinous acts. There is so much to forgive in this world. But remember, our goal is to release resentments from our nervous system so that we can feel positive emotions again. If you are spiritually inclined, you may find great comfort on this topic from a spiritual text translated into over two dozen languages, A Course In Miracles. This text advises us that we don't have to know how to forgive; we just have to be "willing" to forgive. A Course In Miracles assures us that if we are willing to "let go of our suffering," a loving intelligence that connects us all (aka God) will do the heavy lifting of forgiveness. We don't have to feel like forgiveness is a mysterious, arduous process. We just need to want to forgive genuinely. If you are not spiritually inclined, just think about this tool as an opportunity to repro-gram the subconscious mind to release your griev-ances. That works too, right? I have lived this grace personally, and I can vouch that it works! If I find myself constricting my heart area because I am holding on to resentment, I set a sincere intention to release it. Often I notice later that it disappeared, but I never knew exactly when it happened. I just found myself laughing easier again relatively soon. Because I have been training for so long, I will notice much sooner than most when this small miracle has occurred. This tool works nicely for less complicated situations but takes repetition for more serious breaches.

Often, we think of forgiveness as a one-time event, or we believe that we could forgive some things but not others. People are often reluctant to forgive because they feel they let someone "slide" by forgiving them multiple times. They conclude that because they have been disappointed, they have a permanent reason never to forgive them. If we feel we have been wronged numerous times by someone, it is often essential to set emotional boundaries so it does not happen again. However, even if we set boundaries, and they are breached, we need to keep our hearts soft for our benefit. It may be helpful to ruminate on Jesus's answer to Peter's question in the gospel of Matthew. Peter asks Jesus, "How many times should we forgive? Seven times? " And Jesus answered, "Seven times seventy." When biblical scholars performed the numerology for Jesus' statement, they found that Jesus actually meant that we should forgive an infinite number of times. This is an example of how many ancient spiritual traditions are being verified by current neuroscience. As you come to learn just how much we burden ourselves with conscious and unconscious resentments, we understand the wisdom of Jesus's statement. There is no minimally acceptable limit of forgiveness. To become liberated, we need to be forgiving resentments toward others continually, throughout each day, every day, as the 40 years of Zen work objectively demonstrates. Whether it is the wisdom of the sages or current neuroscience, we know that forgiveness is powerful for significantly enhancing the quality of life.

In this mind-body exploration, *Heart Hygiene For*

Emotional Liberation, you will experience a mind-body technique that I call visual forgiveness, which is both simple and laser-like effective. We will combine increasing heart rate variability with the power of focused, mental, cleansing light, until we feel compassion for our perpetrator. No, this is not a spiritual bypass; in fact, it is the exact opposite. It takes a courageous, highly skilled deep dive direct into the deepest hurts lodged in our cell tissue to release them and allow a pearl of greater wisdom to emerge. The rewards of this bravery is experiencing infinitely greater compassion.

The meditation for this chapter will take you through the steps to feel the exquisite freedom of forgiveness, which will often make you crave more of it! I know I am addicted to the release of forgiveness. Resentments make me feel bogged down, and I no longer am willing to tolerate that long term. As my daughter said as a young child, "Forgiveness is fun!" I know you may not believe me yet, but just give it a try. You may get hooked, too! If the word forgiveness is too heavy for you, just think of the phrases emotional release or emotional freedom.

We will begin the meditation by tethering our minds to the energetic heart area in the body and relaxing the chest wall muscles. Then, we will synch breathing with heart rate to induce more heart rate variability. Next, we will invoke the restorative emotions of appreciation, love, and care to anchor into our well-being. The next step will be to remember a resentment and feel where we clutch, grip, or grasp in the body. We often feel grievances as a tightness in the heart area, but not always. In the next chapter, we will discuss how to handle resentment contractions in other parts of the body. Even if we release resentments in other parts of the body, it increases our heart rate variability. However, for the mind-body exploration for this chapter, we will be focusing on releasing the heart. We will take a moment or two to feel this hurt and let it "land" within our heart-center. Directly confronting resentments for situations that hurt us may sound scary, but remember, we would have already invoked heart rate variability to provide emotional stability. Then we will think of our perpetrators and find ways of feeling empathy for them. We will explore many different perspectives to find an angle that enables us to feel great compassion. When we have this compassionate perspective in mind, we will take an emotional snapshot. We will set an intention to remember this person from this loving perspective every time they come to our mind. We will also hold compassion for ourselves to establish healthy boundaries when necessary.

I do believe that we do the best we can with what we have experienced in life. Often, if we knew a better way to get our needs met, we would have done better.

It is often helpful for us to maintain this understanding perspective while considering our transgressors. When we feel compassion for our transgressors, we are finally on our way to exploring the luxurious freedom of forgiveness. Lousy behavior always arises from our insecurities and our lack of confidence that we can meet our own needs. When we view poor behavior from this perspective, it becomes much easier to find the compassion needed to extend forgiveness to others. Once we have compassion for our perpetrator, we will imagine using a cleansing, purifying light to cleanse any residual resentment from the interaction.

Because I have witnessed beautiful results for both myself and others from doing this meditation, I now do a daily practice of it in some form. Nothing has empowered me more in the last few years than variations of this meditation theme. I find it as critical to do every day as brushing my teeth. Just as people would not think of going too long without brushing their teeth, I find that I don't want to allow myself to go too long without doing forgiveness or release work. I have personally had thousands of instances that remind me of this work's power over many years, and my clients report the same benefits as well. Often after doing a forgiveness meditation, I have had disagreements vanish or communications softened without any additional effort.

The forgiveness exploration uses the heart as a biofeedback instrument to determine whether we are in a state of forgiveness. By generating feelings of forgiveness, we will be increasing heart rate variability. This meditation is revolutionary because we will forgive physically and visually, not merely psychologically. Quite frankly, forgiveness does not often make rational sense. However, from the realm of releasing stuck energy of the body, it makes complete sense.

Remember, according to A Course In Miracles; we are not expected to do the heavy work of lifting negativity from our hearts. We are only invited to be "willing" to have the negativity lifted. We don't have to go to therapy for years to forgive. We can just allow resentments to be released from our cell tissue. We will accomplish this by skillfully feeling resentful feelings while increasing heart rate variability and then cleansing our hearts with the power of light (more on the power of light in chapter 6). We need just to be "willing" to let go of suffering. In A Course of Miracles, we are repeatedly asked to have a "little willingness" to forgive, and our subconscious will handle the rest.

Curiously, the heart even helps us to process this work mentally. Heartmath's research also reveals that increased HRV enables cortical facilitation, a mechanism that allows us to shape perceptions of events resourcefully. Basically, that means that when we experience greater heart rate variability more of the time, we are less likely to view troubling situations from a depressing limited point of view. While experiencing cortical facilitation, we review conditions from a resourceful perspective. Remember when I told you that the heart is the most extensive oscillator of the body, and its heartbeat is measured anywhere on the entire body? Your heartbeat influences your brain's functioning as well, so if the heart is not setting off healthy electromagnetic signals, it negatively affects our brain's perceptions

For us to have a well-rounded understanding of this phenomenon, it is helpful to discuss cortical inhibition, the opposite of cortical facilitation. Cortical inhibition is part of the hardwired fight-or-flight mechanism within us, so it is activated when we feel we are in a threatening situation. When we are fearful, it is harder for us to gain the higher cortical function levels to help us make the right decisions. To describe it succinctly, when we are stressed, we just can't think as clearly. Our brain waves become as dysfunctional as our heart rate variability. However, when the heart has a healthy heart rate variability, it synchronizes with our brain waves in a manner that shifts our perceptions toward the positive. This perceptual shift is known as cortical facilitation, and it results in greater clarity and creative thinking. Learning how to encourage cortical facilitation saves unnecessary wear and tear on the body and promotes a positive, healthy balance. It also significantly contributes to our happiness.

Sometimes people think that if they forgive others for transgressions, they will become weak and passive. I have found the exact opposite is true. The more I release and let go of the past, the freer I am to speak my mind. As Gandhi said, "forgiveness is an attribute of the strong." The more we seek to rid ourselves of resentments, even petty jealousies, the stronger we become. We are physically stronger after we forgive. There is an old saying, "forgive, or relive." When we stop squandering our spirit in reliving the past, we have more of our heart available in the present to invest in our lives for the better.

The forgiveness exploration for this chapter will teach you how to bring all these skills and concepts together. It will show you how to pluck resentments that keep a stranglehold on your heart rate variability. If you are interested in purchasing a simple biofeedback instrument that teaches people how to manage their Heart Rate Variability, you can find one on our website at ConsciousnessAthletes.com, or Heartmath.com.

Our Consciousness Athlete program teaches people to maintain open hearts, helping our students be incredibly resilient and buoyant. Nothing in life can get Consciousness Athletes down for long. They know they must choose daily, sometimes over and over and over again, to guard their hearts against life's inevitable betrayals. They refuse to become a slave to any tragedy, and they have the intentional support of the group of other Consciousness Athletes to do that. They know that nothing is more important than keeping their hearts open and being unafraid of loving with abandon. They have conditioned their nervous system for well-being and find that holding grudges is intolerable to them. They know they will energetically wither and diminish if they don't release the toxic drain on their energy. Because they are committed to the Consciousness Athlete work and trust its alchemy, they release resentments knowing they will become more emotionally liberated, which will open many more options for them. This increase in energy gives them more **juice** to feel buoyant and expansive and more sublime feelings of appreciation, love, and courage. They know what it is like to feel "Just gorgeous!" on the inside.

After doing the mind-body *Heart Hygiene for Emotional Liberatio*n exploration, I will ask you to notice how different you feel. Consider this: if you can significantly change your state in such a short amount of time, what would happen if you let go a little bit more every day? How different would you feel by the end of the week? How fabulous would you feel after thirty days? Through this process, we learn an unkept secret. *Buoyant feelings never end!!* We understand that well-being feelings are infinite, so we can become gluttons for love.

The Course In Miracles tells us that "forgiveness is our only function." When I read that phrase years ago, I overlaid my religious training on it. I thought that forgiveness would be our only function because forgiving would enable us to live from pure love. However, throughout my years, I have gained a much broader energetic understanding of these words. I realized that forgiveness is our only function because when we maintain resentments, we lose access to our most precious commodity, our spirit. We need our spirit to be available in the present time to live the whole purpose of our lives. The buoyant feelings that emerge from authentic forgiveness offer us the greatest gift we could ever receive, the creative life force essence of our spirit.

In the next chapter, you will learn how to liberate more of your spirit through body release. When we have access to more of our essential being, we can move into even sweeter places within ourselves. Many of us have had our life force trapped for far too long, significantly diminishing our happiness. Be sure to savor your release thoroughly because you will acclimate to it quickly. The good news is that as your happiness baseline continues to increase, your overall capacity for greater joy rises as well. Think of it as your heart getting bigger which adds greater meaning and joy to your life. Enjoy!

You can find the *Heart Hygiene For Facilitating Emotional Freedom* Exploration at ConsiousnessAthletes.com/explorations.

Enter the password: explore

Enjoy!

Chapter Three Notes:
Conditioning Your Body For Happiness
By Transferring Consciousness Athlete Skills
into Daily Life

Please listen to the mind-body exploration Heart Hygiene For Facilitating Emotional Freedom for this chapter 5 times.

It is virtually impossible for us to feel happy,

when our chest muscles are tight

and we have reduced heart-rate variability.

Many of us live lives of heightened responsibility, which puts our hearts in lockdown, and if left unchecked, reduces our capacity for joy.

There are many seasons of life where we must perform essential duties for long periods. It is during these times that it is even more critical for us to release our hearts daily.

We learn that becoming light-hearted is a worthy endeavor.

Treat your heart like a garden each day.

Pluck it of resentments.

Water it with useful, uplifting information through books, people, or self-soothing activities.

As the poet Georgia Heard suggested,

allow yourself to "fall in love three times a day."

Be sure to imagine a beautiful light shining into your heart area and sense the energy field surrounding your heart expanding (more on that in future chapters).

If something challenging happens, imagine blowing the negativity out of your body like you are blowing on a dandelion and watching the seeds disperse in the air.

Feel the exquisite release of permanently releasing negativity.

Allow yourself to sink into deeper states of well-being. As you release your heart more and more each day, come to understand how love is infinite, and there are no limitations on joy.

Please visit consciousnessathletes.com/explorations

Enter the password: explore

CHAPTER 4 - LOVING AWAY
OUR EMOTIONAL ADDICTIONS

When people start working with me, I make them a promise. I guarantee they will soon find themselves far more fascinating than they ever realized! I promise this because, as we work together, I know they will remember forgotten pockets of meaningful information about who they are that they have been unconsciously stifling. When this suppressed information is revealed, it changes everything! People have a fundamental shift in how they view themselves, which invites them to open doors to a new array of choices and opportunities for their lives.

These shifts are profound, but not because people are discovering something new. They merely remember the truth of who they have always been. As children, we learn to silence aspects of ourselves to conform to our parents' and society's wishes. We are taught to pay more attention to outside directions instead of inside emotional cues. Unfortunately, this social conditioning process causes us to lose the inner compass of our own soul's journey. Through this process, we tragically lose track of our most vital resource: our own soul essence. Making major life decisions without gathering information from our soul's essence often causes us to experience numerous repercussions for decades. We may choose a partner who is not suited to us, invest in an inappropriate career path, or yield to others' expectations, instead of living from our own core set of values.

As you continue to gain the skill of maintaining a conscious presence in your body, you may be bemused and delighted as you start acknowledging activity occurring within you that you have been ignoring for years. Through the Consciousness Athlete training, we learn to acknowledge the infinite number of subtleties occurring within us at every moment. We realize that under our nose is an enormous amount of information emerging from our soul's longings to help us navigate difficult life choices. When we acknowledge and integrate this information, we recognize it provides invaluable insight for navigating our lives in more meaningful and successful ways.

In many traditions, these vital, subtle stirrings are referred to as our heart's wisdom, which reveals our soul. In the previous chapter, we started awakening our souls by clearing our hearts. The heart center is often called "the seat of the soul" because, in many spiritual traditions, the heart is considered the first interface between our physical body and our non-physical soul. Acknowledging the wisdom of your heart, as you did in the mind-body exploration in chapter three, can be considered the first step in honoring your soul's wisdom.

It takes great courage to live from the wisdom of our soul, especially in a world running at such a fast pace that it doesn't even acknowledge we have a soul. Because many of us have not been taught how to interpret the soul's stirrings in our hearts, we snuff them out. It takes great courage to live with heart. In fact, the root of the word courage comes from the Latin word cor, which translates as the word heart. The original word courage meant to speak one's mind by telling all one's heart. Have you ever had to speak up about something that is troubling your heart? If so, you know that it can require great courage. Often, we would rather keep our understandings quiet, instead of rocking the boat. Because many of us have endured significant hardships and traumas, we often ignore our heart's wisdom because we fear that speaking our heart's truth will cause more problems. Undoubtedly, many times in life, we may need to quell our heart's truth. However, as a blanket life strategy, this practice spells disaster for both our health and happiness.

Shamanic practices recognize the repercussions of living without heart. Shamans—indigenous medical doctors—work with sick patients from a very different perspective than Western medical doctors. Shamans believe we become unwell when we hemorrhage our heart's power. According to shamanic traditions, when we are not living life anchored in our hearts, we lose personal power, resulting in physical illness and complicated life circumstances. Shamans believe that a portion of our soul may leave our body during stressful situations, resulting in physical and emotional illness. Symptoms of soul loss include physical illness, feelings of depression, lack of clarity, loss of self-control, and feeling that a portion of yourself died after experiencing an especially difficult time. From a Shamanic perspective, when we experience such internal turmoil, our spirit needs healing, not just our physical body.

Remember my description of the rising pitch of the Galvanic Skin Response (GSR) biofeedback instrument, when people's awareness ascends the body while talking about their stress? Because of my experience with shamanic traditions, I've often wondered if this GSR phenomenon is the shamanic equivalent of a person's soul leaving their body. Based on my repeated observations regarding healing over the years through biofeedback instrumentation, I believe there is some truth to the shamanic understanding of soul loss. My experience studying EEG Neurofeedback with Judith Pennington, the world's authority on the Mind Mirror EEG instrument, also supported my observations. Judith studies advanced meditators at the Monroe Institute, the premier and internationally known research organization for out-of-body soul travel. These are individuals who have trained themselves to allow their consciousness to disassociate from their bodies skillfully. Judith has reviewed the brainwave patterns of people who expertly train their spirit to leave their bodies to explore consciousness and beyond.

Most of us experience our sense of self inside our physical bodies. Most view the world around us from this vantage point, as well. But during an out-of-body experience (OBE), people can observe themselves from outside of themselves, looking in. They see the world from a much more fluid, expansive perspective. Many people at the Monroe Institute demonstrate their top-notch skill by identifying the hidden object's location during their out-of-body excursions.

Judith and others have documented a signature EEG pattern on the Mind Mirror instrument of a person who has left his or her body. Interestingly, the brainwave signal's amplitude, which is often on average at least eight microvolts, will reduce to virtually zero microvolts in four of the five brainwave categories. Think about that! I mean, for comparison, brain death is demonstrated by all of the brainwave amplitudes reducing to zero microvolts. These EEG biofeedback measurements support my conclusions about the GSR measurements that consciousness does leave the body at times, whether people are aware of it or not.

The Monroe Institute meditators have trained to come into command of their ability to leave the body, so they are doing it safely and with a broad knowledge base of experience. However, it is common for people in daily life to experience trauma and have their consciousness spontaneously leave their bodies without their knowledge. Psychologists refer to this phenomenon as a "dissociative" experience. I have spent over two decades clinically observing people connected to GSR as they undergo emotional and physical healings. In general, the more centered and balanced people feel, the easier it is for them to maintain awareness in their bodies. When people are feeling whole and complete, they keep the pitch of the GSR low and stable. As I observe this phenomenon daily, I get a palpable sense that as people bring their awareness down into the body, a portion of their soul becomes present that was not there just a few moments earlier. If you are interested in working with a GSR at home, please visit our website: ConsciousnessAthletes.com. The GSR will offer you palpable feedback regarding the infinite subtle activity that is occurring within you. Tapping this information could provide valuable information for your life.

According to shamanic tradition, we can "lose" a portion of our soul if we undergo a traumatic experience. The soul part will often return on its own. However, problems occur when individuals are no longer able to call their souls back home to their physical bodies. That is when shamans intervene, to retrieve soul essence. To help retrieve the soul part, shamans are taught to move their awareness into a deep, loving space that holds no judgment for the patient. The shaman then "journeys back in time" to retrieve the patient's soul parts and then reunites them with the patient's spirit.

There are times in life when we may experience a breach of our soul, and not even know it. As we continue living our lives without a portion of our essence, we may find ourselves in monotonous daily struggles. We may repeat unhealthy patterns, get lost in addictions, experience frequent depressions, feel haunted by fears of unworthiness or struggle with insomnia. You may not remember when the soul loss started, or you may know precisely when it happened because you remember something fundamentally shifted within yourself after the event. The good news is that the work of this book and its accompanying mind-body explorations is a version of soul retrieval that will help you restore your spirit back to its original fullness. When we set a firm intention to anchor our mind in the body, it is similar to the shamanic tradition of calling our spirit back into the body. As we practice these skills, we become happier because we have more of our spirit in the present time to finance our lives.

Maintaining the integrity of our spirit is important because it is the fuel that finances our lives. If our spirit is trapped in old stories, we live life in "economy mode." We don't have the energy in our system to confront familiar struggles or take on the challenge of establishing new habits. When we anchor our mind in the body, our brain's default mode network, responsible for most of our suffering, finally turns off. We become free to experience the purity of the moment without a story overlay. As we gain greater access to our spirit, new doors open within ourselves, resulting in a flourishing of health and creativity. My team and I witness these transformations repeatedly when people participate in Global Peaceful City Projects, sponsored by the non-profit I founded, NUMINOUS. As participants skillfully move their nervous system into a feeling of greater love and wholeness, they gain new perspectives. These insights give them the strength and inspiration to start new creative projects.

This state of wholeness has undeniably palpable benefits. It is not whimsical, ephemeral, or vague.

With training, it becomes a reliable, familiar place within ourselves. We learn to tune our inner world, similar to how we would tune a guitar to play a beautiful song. We become highly skilled at recognizing when we are present and when we are not. When we acknowledge that we are not present, we have the skills to move our mind's awareness into the body, relax the area that is constricted, and let it go. As we let go physically, we simultaneously learn how to let go emotionally. At first, our mental patterns may be so well-entrenched, we find it extremely difficult to stop clutching the body when we think of our stressors. However, with training, we become skilled at remaining calm in our bodies as we review challenges. Eventually, we realize that an over-activated default mode network is not worth the agony. We come to understand that maintaining an awareness of the ground state of being is far more enjoyable than the endless drama created by the rumination caused by our rambling default mode network.

There is currently an explosion of research being conducted that is studying rumination, the process of continuously thinking about the same thoughts, which tend to be sad or dark. The habit of rumination can be dangerous. In her book, Women Who Think Too Much, Susan Nolen-Hoeksema discusses how women, especially, often ruminate over the losses in their lives. They go round and round in their minds, overthinking, and repeatedly ask themselves why people acted as they did. They can waste decades of their lives trying to make sense of things that will never make sense. To silence these endless ruminations, they often try to mood alter through alcoholism, eating disorders, or other substance abuse. I have personally witnessed family members terrorize themselves with these mental patterns, literally until their death. The tyranny of the mind can be so severe I find it heartbreaking. I have come to understand why so many people resort to substance abuse to eliminate their suffering. Most people just don't have the tools that provide the grit required to stop ruminating. The exploration for this chapter offers the mind-body skills to set yourself free.

To begin exploring this soul recovery process, read this text slowly as you take a moment to scan your body from head to toe. Feel the space above your head, the surface beneath your feet. Become aware of the space to the left of you and to the right of you. Become mindful of how you are sitting on the chair or lying on the bed. Become aware of the space three hundred and six degrees around your body. Imagine that there is a sphere of light surrounding your body. Feel your breathing. Turn inward. You may want to close your eyes and pause for a moment to take an assessment of how you feel before you read the next paragraph.

Now, bring to mind your life's biggest challenge. Where in your body do you clutch, grip, or grasp? Take a moment and move your awareness into the area. Notice that when you review this challenge, this specific part of your body contracts. If you were to do this over a period of time, you would notice how this contraction is highly precise and consistent. So, what is happening there? The flow of life force in your body stops in that part of your body every time you think the same thought. In fact, until the challenging energy is authentically reconciled, that part of your body will always contract in that exact location.

Let's take a moment to understand what is happening. The more we clutch at that area, the less our spirit is free to move toward resolution. On the energetic level, and even often at the muscular level, our spirit is actually stuck. As we have been learning, when our spirit is bound in emotional issues, we cannot use the energy to finance our lives, which robs us of our joy.

Let's try this again so that you gain a broader understanding. Read this text slowly to keep your mind's awareness with your body. Again, relax and calm your body by sinking into the surface beneath you. Become aware of the space three hundred and sixty degrees around your body. Feel your feet beneath you and become aware of the area above your head and body. Feel your breathing and turn inward. Now think of a different challenge in your life. Pause for a moment as you scan your body. Where do you feel your body tightening when you consider this challenge?

Most people will contract in an entirely different location when they consider this second issue. Isn't that interesting? As we review various challenges in our lives, we contract different parts of our body. Contracting is our instinctive response as we attempt to protect ourselves from emotional pain. We stop the flow of emotional energy, which keeps us from feeling overwhelmed. Please understand that physical muscular contractions are adaptive mechanisms that enable us to survive, or even thrive, despite the challenges we face. If you find a place of contraction, understand that it is your body's way of protecting you.

However, when we are no longer in control of these muscular contraction patterns, it could be said that we have an emotional addiction. Our chronic unconscious emotional ruminations create predictable muscular bracing patterns that are beyond our conscious control. We become so accustomed to feeling the constriction that, like any other addiction, it becomes extremely complicated to stop. We become attached to a particular internal environment that accompanies a chronic struggle. We may think there is no way out, or that we have to live with this emotional pain for the rest of our lives. Sadly, we often don't even realize we are responsible for constricting the area of life force, hence our pain. We then often berate ourselves for having such a hard time getting over life's challenges. Here is the big secret that too few people know: it is easier to break emotional addictions when you become conscious of your chronic muscular patterns. When we release the body's specific part that tightens as we review challenges, we accelerate our ability to resolve them! There is a key out of our personal prison, and it is hidden in plain sight!

I have presented this topic to large groups for twenty-five years. I never tire of asking audiences where they grip when they consider their life's most significant issue. Audience members will share that they tighten in their heart, abdomen, or shoulders; others may say they contract their knees, jaw, or head. When people share where they contract, everyone learns that everyone's stress response is different. Not everyone tightens their abdomen when they talk about their greatest challenge. Some people tighten their left knee's back, furrow their right eyebrow, or clench their hands or jaw.. I find these differences between people fascinating.

I also ask people if they find they are clutching in an area associated with a health condition they experience. More often than not, the places where participants are clutching are the precise locations related to their health challenges. For instance, someone with high blood pressure may feel gripping in their heart area. Someone who has had back surgeries will clutch the same location in their back where they had surgery. The place I have found the most intriguing has been the throat. More often than not, when people feel gripping in their throat, they take medicine for a malfunctioning thyroid! Recently, a young woman told me she found herself gripping in her throat when she considered her life challenge. I told her, "Well, if you were older, I would ask you if you are on thyroid medication." She replied, "I am!" Even I was shocked at the correlation.

This experience drove home to me the potential negative consequences of emotional addictions. Chronic emotional clutching patterns can have a dramatic negative impact on our health. As we gain a deep understanding of this phenomenon, we can appreciate the wisdom of the shamanic soul retrieval perspective. When you perform the mind-body exploration for this chapter, be sure to note if your clutching areas correspond with your health challenges. If not, I would like to think that you will still be avoiding health issues by doing the Consciousness Athlete work. Your emotional addiction may not be associated with a health issue at this point, but if it kept progressing, it could. My clinical observations have led me to believe that unattended emotional addictions could be similar to smoking, where we don't feel the negative consequences until decades later. If chronic emotional habits are left unattended over time, they cause long term wear and tear on the body.

In this mind-body exploration, we will practice contemplating emotional challenges while maintaining body release in the affected areas. For many of you, this will not be easy. It will feel like a mental tongue twister. Please be kind to yourself! You have been chronically tightening this area for so long that you probably lost conscious control of it a long time ago. As we learn to relax while contemplating a challenging issue, we access a much more significant portion of our spirit offering us a greater perspective. We gain an enlightened detachment, one that enables us to honor the struggle's complexity, instead of being frightened by it. Even if it feels challenging to keep this area released as you review the tough issue, keep at it! Because an inherent dignity will eventually arise from deep within due to your hard work, and it is liberating!

There is another tool we will be adding to this mind-body exploration to hone our focusing skills. Instead of just using our focus like a neutral lazer, we will alter our focus to beam a nourishing, unconditional, loving presence to the contracted area. With this loving focus, we will honor our struggles and love ourselves for our attempts to resolve them. We will come to peace within ourselves, which is reflected in our relaxed body. This emancipation will take some practice. People are most successful at learning how to release chronic contractions while they are in the lower brain waves of relaxation produced during meditation. The brainwaves you are in now while reading this book are not very conducive for you to embrace this loving state.

There are specific physical markers that occur when our body is in a loving state, and meditation helps us feel that love. Blood flows out of large muscles and into the periphery of our hands and feet. Respiration slows down, and our eyes relax. Muscles relax, and the body becomes "doughy." These are all signs that the body has moved into the autonomic nervous system's parasympathetic branch, the part of the nervous system responsible for healing and renewal. When we are in "love," we are being healed genuinely. The more we can maintain a state of loving awareness, the more healed and whole we feel. Advanced Consciousness Athletes strive to perpetually practice maintaining loving internal environments by cultivating open hearts and expanded energy fields. They develop a positive addiction to this state with practice because they have learned how good it feels!

Another advanced skill we will be learning in this mind-body exploration is becoming aware of the space in front and around the body at the site of contraction. There is a field of energy that surrounds our body, often referred to as the Human Biofield or Energy Field. Biofeedback instruments work because we measure changes in this field around the body through electrodes and sensors. Psychics and mediums have been acknowledging the biofield since the beginning of time; however, current western science has been slow to accept it. Albert Szent-Gyorgyi, the 1937 Nobel Prize Winner in Medicine, noted this irony when he said, "In every culture and in every medical tradition before ours, healing was accomplished by moving energy." Finally, the acceptance of insurance for acupuncture and the opportunity for medical professionals to collect continuing education credits for studying energy healing modalities, such as reiki and therapeutic touch, demonstrates that mainstream medicine is now acknowledging the body's energy field. Although many alternative health modalities can help you expand your energy field, and I would recommend many of them, there is nothing more economical than learning how to alter your subtle energy fields through the power of your own mind.

It is accepted in many healing traditions that our spirit's health is reflected in the integrity of our body's energy field. In the mind-body exploration for this chapter, we will be using your honed mental focus to influence your physical body and fortify your spirit by affecting your body's surrounding energy field. Remember when I told you that you will find yourself far more fascinating than you ever realized? Now, you are starting to understand why. This approach will open an infinite realm of new information that can be utilized to improve your health and happiness.

Because you have been cultivating skills developed in the previous chapters, I can finally succinctly summarize how these skills ensure enduring happiness. Essentially, when we are miserable, we have heavy hearts, contracted energy, and tense muscles. When we are happy, our heart feels light, our spirit is anchored and spacious, and our body is released. After all this skill-building, it really comes down to these three parameters. It is so NOT rocket science. There is no mystery to this process. In fact, it is very binary, meaning one of two options, either/or. After gaining mastery of these skills, it becomes clearly evident why happiness has far less to do with what is happening outside of us, like we were taught. Retraining the mind-body connection to be happy is simple and straightforward, but not effortless, which is why many of us need to become Consciousness Athletes if we are to overcome years of negative programming. I'll reiterate the premise of this book:

we are learning how to train the body to sustain happiness, similar to how traditional athletes condition the body for sport. As Consciousness Athletes, we commit to conditioning our body-mind-spirit to remain light, energetically expanded, and muscularly free, even in the face of challenge. Like any other athlete, we must hone our skills and practice to acquire proficiency through difficult challenges.

The mind-body explorations are designed to offer you the necessary inspiration and feedback so you can sustain consistent effort, over time, to condition your body for happiness. The skills you are learning in the mind-body explorations can also be relied upon to manage daily difficult moments, not just when you are meditating. When life challenges you, use your new internal, conscious, athletic ability to move your awareness inward and apply some of your learning skills. You will find that this internal work offers you many more resources—that were hidden previously—to navigate outer circumstances more effectively. Because of our newfound power to shift internally, we learn to become intolerant of feeling miserable over time. Our mind-body explorations have taught us to strive to feel dignity and honor, even during the most challenging times.

When we cultivate the sweet states of well-being, no matter what challenges we are facing, we always remember we can fall up. Through the mind-body explorations, we learn to raise the bar on how good we expect to feel, so we are never entirely willing to surrender our mood to life's circumstances again. We strive to keep our spirit healthy and intact, and we become unwilling to give up our power to anyone or anything. As we practice this state of dignity and honor within us, greater integrity surfaces. This integrity feels like a familiar memory, seeming to come from somewhere far away, yet it feels intimate.

As we learn to maintain the integrity of our inner space, we remember that every challenge is a valuable part of our life's journey. We come to realize that challenges offer us precious opportunities to call back our essential soul. When we have called back enough of our essential soul, we start to feel a deep-welled joy, even during the most difficult moments of our lives. It is often at those challenging moments, we see our progress. We come to a deep appreciation of how the consistent effort we invested in ourselves to become a consciousness athlete is paying us back in spades.

Please access the mind-body exploration Loving Away Our Emotional Addictions at ConsciousnessAthletes.com

Enter the password: explore

Chapter Four Notes:
Conditioning Your Body For Happiness
By Transferring Consciousness Athlete Skills
into Daily Life

Please listen to the mind-body exploration Loving Away Our Emotional Addictions for this chapter 5 times.

What is that thing you do that keeps you from being happy?

Think about feeling happy and then noticing what keeps you from allowing happiness to grow within your body?

Where is the hesitation to feel good located in your body?

Now move your kind awareness into that area, and imagine letting the contraction go, similar to how you would feel if you were to open your palm to feel the emptiness of space around it.

How would you live your life differently if you could release that area of your body permanently? What would pure happiness feel like in your body? What different choices would you make?

Set an intention right now to release this area of your body permanently.

Practice releasing this part of your body dozens of times a day, until you catch yourself with the area released without having to prompt yourself.

As you strive to release the restrictions, allow joy, contentment, openness, or spaciousness to take its place.

Please
visit consciousnessathletes.com/explorations

Enter the password: explore

CHAPTER 5 - EXPANSIVE STATES FOR HIGHER STAKES

Did you ever feel like there was a limit to how happy you can feel? Do you walk around waiting for "the other shoe to drop?" Have you ever felt delighted in a particular environment, but the moment you left the situation, your spirit sagged, and stale old negative stories about your flaws flared? Conversely, have you ever felt sick and in pain, but then something made you laugh, and suddenly, you felt so good and your pain levels dropped? Have you ever *consciously challenged these fluctuations in your spirit*? Wouldn't it be great if you did not have to descend into low emotions after feeling incredible highs?

Three people's work has given me great insight into how to use emotional fluctuations as rudders, leading to more joyful states. After learning how they made skillful choices that escalated their joy, I have integrated their work as I created biofeedback tools for the Consciousness Athlete curriculum. My program takes the guesswork out of establishing happiness within ourselves. I guarantee that if you perform this work consistently and well, you will always lift your spirit. I can offer this promise because you will be releasing the very restrictions that keep buoyant, good feelings at bay. This curriculum goes far beyond simply helping you experience more pleasure in the current moment. It also primes you to increase your capacity for more joy each day. Teaching this work, I see that people are exceptionally grateful to find it offers such a straight path toward happiness and fulfillment. Following this curriculum enables us to feel a sense of accomplishment and track our progress.

In the years before I created this curriculum, I often felt curious and perplexed about fluctuations in my own emotions. However, I then experienced a period during which I could no longer afford even the slightest emotional change. Years ago, before the winter holidays, I experienced a tragedy so significant that it even appeared in the local news for several weeks. The emotional pain was so bad at times that my knees would buckle as I walked due to high levels of cortisol released in my system. One evening, my children were away with their father for the holidays, and I was home alone, managing my shattered heart. I awoke at 3:00 AM, feeling the excruciating ache in my body-mind. To ease the pain, I decided to get up and work on my first website for the Global Peaceful Cities Project.

As I worked, I thought about the peace project's transformative consciousness athlete meditation skills and how lucky I was to have them to strengthen me during my darkest days. I contemplated how the website's skills could help others like me facing tragedy at 3:00 AM. These emotional survival skills helped me function through devastating loss—I didn't want anyone else to suffer disabling grief without them. The more I thought about how sharing these skills would help people through their worst days, the happier I became, and the more blessed I felt. I started working with greater zeal. But then I began to question myself: "What was I genuinely feeling? Which feelings was I feeling?" From feeling devastating loss, I had moved toward tasting the sweet nectar of service. How could I feel so genuinely happy when my eyes were still bloodshot from crying? Startlingly, I felt so strong, resilient, and happy, within mere moments of feeling weak, devastated, and crushed. How could that possibly be? I was experiencing the greatest loss of my life, but I felt whole and complete.

In the weeks that followed, I often felt I was walking a razor's edge between these contrasting emotions. I quickly learned I had to actively stay in my wholeness, or I would become devoured by dreadful details, unleashing a cascade of anxiety crippling stress hormones. Because the feeling of wholeness was such a life raft for emotional stability during this time, I learned to be curious about that state of wholeness. What made the difference? How could I be completely fine one moment and struggling the next moment, just to keep myself together?

I noticed that both states presented entirely different experiences in the body. When I felt whole, my shoulders were up and back, my walk was confident, and my eyes focused ahead. My body was more relaxed overall. However, during times of high anxiety, my whole body felt tight. Muscles clutched, gripped, and grasped all over my body, but especially in my abdomen. Life is the the most outstanding teacher, and this experience offered me an infinite amount of profound lessons. To manage these drastic state changes, I would spend hours meditating with a pillow under my mid-back, to break up the muscular patterns of anxiety in my abdomen. I knew that to be strong enough to work and take care of my young children, I needed to maintain an unwavering state of wholeness.

Many of us go through similar fluctuations of emotions, all day, every day. However, when there is less contrast between the range of our feelings, we are aware of far less feedback from the body, so we don't even acknowledge them. We typically don't notice these fluctuating states. When we do, unfortunately, we often feel powerless to change their direction. Unaware of the inextricable link between emotional states and physical feelings, we are "numb below the ears." We have no idea of the range of emotions we are feeling. This lack of awareness keeps us from noticing that we were holding our breath before our panic attack, which caused the panic attack! Unaware of our breath-holding, we are unable to terminate the panic through proper breathing.

Being unconscious about body cues can also lead to unnecessary stress. For example, arguments can escalate because we missed a signal of increasing frustration: when our hands started clenching. If we had noticed the anger escalating in our body, we might have been able to relax our fists to help us think more clearly, avoiding an argument before it happened. Without body awareness, we don't realize that we have the power to effectively stop feelings of victimization in our mind, only by altering how our bodies feel.

To help you experience this phenomenon, take a moment as you are reading to become aware of your body in space. Become aware of the front and back of your body. Now, become aware of the left and right sides of your body. Feel the top of your head with your awareness, and the bottoms of both feet as well.

Pause for a moment and simultaneously become aware of your entire body and even the space around your body. See if you can exhale fully and let go of any residual tension. Now take a second breath, and let go again.

Now, bring to mind your most significant stressor, and scan your body again. Where are you clutching, gripping, and gasping? Understand that this issue "lives" in that place where your body grips. Each time you think about that stressor, that specific area tightens, so if you want to change how you feel about a situation, relax the area of your body that clutches when you think about it. You may want to put the book down and give that a try right now. Think of the same challenge, but relax in the same area that you just identified. You may want to imagine "sending" your breath into the area to help it stay open and released.

Relaxing this area will take great courage for some of you because you have chronically contracted the area for so long, it may feel uncomfortable to release the space.Allow yourself to feel the pleasurable sensations of release as you let go. Notice how the pain and angst diminishes, and a tender, velvety space emerges. This tender space is critically important because it is the beginning of allowing yourself to bask in sweet emotions again. This pure skill that we may take for granted and often overlook entirely is the precise key that unlocks the door to your joy. When you relax that area for many of you, you will notice that you feel significantly better about the situation. Almost all of us feel better when the body releases, and yet we have emotional habits that maintain our bodies in chronic gripping patterns.

While I was healing from my calamity, this contrast between gripping and release was so stark; it was the difference between me being a competent professional or an emotional puddle! In our regular daily lives, we are undergoing these shifts all day long. Because the consequences are not as severe, we don't even notice the opportunity to improve our emotional weather significantly.

Now become aware of the same area in your body again. Have you been able to keep it relaxed, or do you find yourself gripping still? If you find that space is contracting again, this is where you can start gaining skill in becoming a Consciousness Athlete. In the meditation for this chapter, we will be learning how to condition your body to maintain this opening, similar to the way athletes condition their bodies for endurance sports. Keeping this area released will be identical to most athletic endeavors: it will take practice and repetition to become competent.

If you find yourself continually contracting an area of your body and unable to stop, this is a form of emotional addiction. We get "hooked" to the emotion that causes us to contract that part of the body. In fact, like any addiction, when we try to stop, we may feel a little defeated and lost. That initial, soft opening may feel vulnerable, which some people may interpret as uncomfortable. If this is the case for you, please stick with it. Strive to find some compassionate courage for yourself, and reclaim control of that part of your body and mind. I have combed my body with my mind, searching for contracting spaces within myself, for many years. I don't find nearly as many of these pockets left within me anymore, reflecting my elevated mood baseline. However, if I do discover areas where I grip, I strive to release them immediately. I meet the challenge, knowing that I am reclaiming a portion of my spirit back into the present. I am no longer willing to subconsciously surrender my power to the situation and have my cell tissue pay for it.

This state of wholeness is not something ephemeral, fleeting, or vague. With training, it becomes a reliable place within ourselves. We learn to tune our inner world, similar to how we would need to tune a neglected guitar to play a beautiful song. We become highly skilled at recognizing when we are present and when we are not. When we acknowledge that we are not present, we move our awareness into the body, relax the constricted area, and release it. As we let go physically, we are learning how to let go emotionally.

Because our emotional addictions are so entrenched within the fabric of our spirit, we may find this extremely difficult to accomplish at first. However, with training over time, we become highly skilled at returning home to our bodies. Eventually, we realize that the pain of "leaving our body" and activating the default mode network (DMN) is not worth the agony. Maintaining an awareness of our state of being is far more desirable than the drama of our rambling DMN, with its accompanying muscle contractions.

We can observe this powerful process in the lives of three extraordinary people, who made the trek from fluctuating agony to permanent bliss, and, the best part is, they left a trail of breadcrumbs for us to follow. Lester Levenson, Peace Pilgrim, and Brother Lawrence were each intolerant of feeling miserable within their difficult circumstances. Making happiness their mission, they refused to settle for anything less. They demonstrate that we should not settle for unhappiness either, because, with a disciplined mind, we all have access to heightened states of being. Through relentless mental focus, they willed themselves to increase their joy, even during tough situations. Using their difficulties as pivot points for elevating their consciousness, they became outliers of extreme happiness. Their writings documented their journeys into joy. Although they all came from modest and often difficult means, all three died exceptionally happy people. They are my heroes. In this book, I have created a dynamic combination that I have never seen recorded anywhere else. I combined the mental influences of Brother Lawrence, Peace Pilgrim, and Lester Levinson

with my combination of palpable concrete biofeedback skills *intertwined* with subtle energy expansion skills to ensure and accelerate all of our success. Based on my elevated mood trajectory and our research, I will discuss in chapter six, I'm 100% confident that I will eventually die in a similar sweet state, as well.

One common theme of their lives was their extraordinary willingness to let go of negative emotions. Each had the mental acuity to discern which emotions lead to greater happiness and which emotions lead to debilitating pain. Like to my story, they reached a point in their lives where they were no longer willing to tolerate feeling miserable. Unwilling to ruminate on negativity, they experienced the natural swelling of good feelings by learning to skillfully release their bodies, which in turn, liberated their minds.

We will begin with Lester Levinson, an exceptionally bright physicist, successful businessman, and self-made millionaire. Although he had experienced impressive success by the world's standards, he suffered from inner turmoil. At the age of 42, Lester had his second massive heart attack. Bypass surgery and heart transplants were not available at that time, so when he came out of the emergency room, the doctors said, "Lester, we're sorry to tell you, but you have two weeks to live, three at the most, and we can't do anything for you. So we're sending you home." Lester went home and realized that he did not know much at all because he was so miserable despite his considerable academic and worldly knowledge. This revelation started him on an intense examination of his life.

Lester observed every fluctuating emotion he ever had. He noticed that each time he was ill, he wanted something, and these intense feelings of want were making him miserable. Lester realized he wanted love. He wanted money. He wanted to change things. Whenever he craved something, he had an uncomfortable feeling that could be traced back to his illness. Then he had another realization. Reminiscing about the love he felt for his former girlfriend, he suddenly felt right. Eventually, he realized that he was not ill whenever he was giving, loving, and not wanting anything.

Illness can provide powerful emotional feedback. When the body is so compromised, something that causes relief feels magnified, so it can easily be associated with happiness and contentment. Lester was astute enough to notice this stark contrast, and he also had a strong enough will to propel himself forward.

Lester eventually asked himself a big question: "if I could get rid of all my non-loving feelings, would I heal?" He went on a vigorous quest to eliminate all negative feelings, striving to feel only love. He challenged himself to search his consciousness for anything that made him less happy and continue thinking about it until he felt only love! He became so addicted to feeling love—it felt so good, so sweet, and so perfect—that he believed it to be the only state of being from which he wanted to live.

Eventually, Lester made another discovery: when he was loving, he was happiest. That happiness equated to being loving rather than being loved. He started wondering if he could cure his illnesses this way, so he started using his will to direct all of his thoughts from "wanting to be loved" to that of "loving." Examining all his relationships, he let go of all of his non-loving feelings from the past.

During this process, Lester realized he had formerly wanted to change the entire world to meet his preferences. His desire for control had been the cause of all his ailments. His opinionated preferences were making him a slave to this world. He decided to reverse this tendency by unloading all-controlling subconscious concepts and pressures and taking responsibility for everything happening in his life. Recognizing that his mental patterns were the source of his problems, he simultaneously realized they were limitations he could quickly drop.

Eventually, he came to believe good feelings are the infinite essence of God within us and that every person has access to infinite, divine love, with no limitations. With this last realization, he became even happier: freer and lighter, with an overall sense of expansive well-being. Lester learned how to hack his well-being by understanding how our mind can create either misery or mastery. According to the adage, "The mind is a wonderful servant but a terrible master," Lester spent the remainder of his life helping others discover this secret of self-mastery. He shared his teachings of the Sedona method until he passed at the age of 84—42 years after being told he had only two to three weeks to live!

Three aspects to Lester's story are important to elucidate here, because you will see these same traits in the next two examples. First, Lester found himself in a miserable place and then discovered a pocket of relief when he noted how good it feels to offer love. Second, he had a strong will! It was the same will that made him such an enormously successful business-man. As a self-made man, Lester embraced self-responsibility. That same willingness to follow his relentless will skillfully guided him out of turmoil. He never gave up, even when he expected to live only two to three weeks. His pain became his springboard because he was unwilling to wallow in his sorrow. Third, as Peace Pilgrim and Brother Lawrence, he landed in the understanding that there is an infinite loving divine presence within each of us. They all independently discovered that living poised from that point of reference was an unparalleled joy.

Peace Pilgrim followed a similar course, experiencing the same unbounded happiness. Formerly known as Mildred Lisette Norman, Peace was an American non-denominational spiritual teacher and peace activist. She vowed to "remain a wanderer until mankind has learned the way of peace, walking until I am given shelter and fasting until I am given food." Peace Pilgrim walked across the United States for 28 years, touching thousands of hearts, minds, and spirits through her message of inner peace. She was on her seventh cross-country journey when she died. Peace Pilgrim walked in complete peace, confident that her basic needs would be met at all times. "I don't even ask," Peace said, "it's given without asking. I tell you, people are good. There's a spark of good in everybody." Peace was the "real deal." How many 73-year-olds do you know who are happy sleeping under bridges after walking for days in the elements? Peace was a walking demonstration of how to use the power of our will to live from buoyant states. States that feel so whole and complete, we are happy to hold on to nothing.

Peace did not begin her life from such pursuits. As a young woman, she followed the latest trends. Peace Pilgrim's sister, Helene Young, says Mildred "was very much what they called a flapper in those days. She had to have the latest clothing." However, these material pursuits soon bored Peace. As she wrote in her booklet, *Steps Toward Inner Peace*,

> *In my early life, I made two very important discoveries. In the first place, I discovered that making money was easy. And in the second place, I discovered that making money and spending it foolishly was completely meaningless. I knew that this was not what I was here for. And so I went into the second phase of my life. I began to live to give what I could, instead of get what I could, and I entered a new and wonderful world. My life began to become meaningful. I attained the great blessing of good health; I haven't had a cold or headache since. However, there's a great deal of difference between being willing to give your life, and actually giving your life, and for me, 15 years of preparation and of inner seeking lay between.*

Peace outlined the four preparations, purifications, and relinquishments she had undergone to reach her state of peace and happiness. She prepared her life of significant meaning by assuming healthy attitudes and beliefs, learning her place in the life pattern, and simplifying her life to reflect her beliefs. She also went through a purification process, where she cleansed her body, thoughts, desires, and motives of unhealthy patterns.

Peace's inner peace did not come "cheap." She struggled during these 15 years as she learned to let go of small, limiting feelings. Similar to Lester Levenson, Peace speaks of how she realized that her negative feelings were hurting her. She understood what psychologists refer to as ego and conscience, the two distinct selves, natures, or wills, with two different viewpoints. Peace recognized that her struggles stemmed from the differing values of these two viewpoints. Complete liberation required her to relinquish the feelings and thoughts associated with her ego.

First, she relinquished her feelings of self-will, the desires of her small self. I know this sounds complicated, but Peace simplifies this step: "it's as though you have two selves: the lower self that usually governs you selfishly, and the higher self which stands ready to use you gloriously. You must subordinate the lower self by refraining from doing the not-good things you are motivated toward, not suppressing them but transforming them so that the higher self can take over your life." Peace goes on to suggest that we redirect the impetus that energizes us toward the "wrong" thing, toward doing the "right" thing. According to Peace, the relinquishment of self-will immediately brings inner peace.

This releasing of the lower self does not sound like much fun at first. With biofeedback and subtle energy practice, it soon becomes clear why it is such a highly desirable state. Feel your self-will in your body when you think about accomplishing something through mental force. How does it feel when you are muscularly clutching to a thought of struggle? Not much fun, right? We feel like we are in a muscular bind. We feel trapped and unhappy with ourselves. As unpleasant as it is not to have our way all the time, feeling this unnecessary discomfort in the face of difficulties is no fun, either. Challenges are already difficult. Why add to them with extreme self-will?

When Peace discusses letting go of the lower self, she refers to releasing the body and the mind. We can't release the mind without releasing the body. This internal release ultimately enables us to feel far greater peace than trying to maintain the impossible task of controlling our world. By controlling her mind, Peace controlled what she experienced through her body. And she was entirely in control of her body: she would command herself to sleep wherever she was, whether on park benches, under bridges, or in fields. This physical mastery is direct proof of Peace's mental prowess.

Peace also relinquished feelings of separateness.

Peace writes, "You can only find harmony when you realize the oneness of all and work for the good of all." Most existential pain stems from feeling separate from our fellow human beings and an infinitely loving source. As the influential spiritual text, *A Course In Miracles*, tells us, we believe we have many problems. However, we have only one problem: the feeling of separateness from an infinite loving intelligence that created us all. When we do the meditation for this chapter, we will release resentments that constrict our bodies to allow more space within us for feeling connected to a greater whole. We will invite our bodies to contact wholeness and love, where we were feeling fear and loss. As we soften the periphery of our body, we release feelings of separateness. We remember how to feel connected to the whole.

As you are learning, we do not tend to go willingly on this journey in the beginning. We have the unproductive habit of identifying with our losses, so it takes an act of will for us to release our suffering. We often have to be just plain tired of the suffering of separateness to finally be willing to "let go" into infinite love. However, once we become comfortable with this process and experience its profound benefits, soon we start looking for additional issues to release so that we can leap into even greater levels of well-being. The day before she died, Peace was a guest on a radio show, and the interviewer commented on Peace's exuberant energy, saying, "She appears to be a most happy woman." Peace Pilgrim responded, "Who could know God and not be joyous?"

Peace also admonished us to relinquish our attachments, which can sound horrible to the modern material mind. But releasing attachment at the nervous system level not mean selling all your stuff and putting your kids up for adoption! You can stay just where you are, with all of your creature comforts, and still live without attachment. Releasing attachments simply means removing the clutching, gripping, and grasping in your nervous system, so that you can walk in pure freedom and joy.

Peace did not suggest that we don't pursue goals. Rather, that we choose our plans wisely, following them with a sense of light playfulness and exploration, rather than relentless drive and compulsion. It is essential to understand that as we release attachments in our energy field, we fill that space with more juice from our own Spirit. So, as we empty ourselves of our clutch on external things, we become more full of our own energy, creativity, and essence! That's how it works. Because these fantastic benefits of releasing attachments are not widely discussed, the practice gets a bum rap. People need to know that releasing attachments actually unearth hidden treasures! It creates a powerful opportunity for our own essential being, with all of its nourishing sweetness, to emerge.

As we release attachments, we understand our unhealthy relationships with our possessions, relationships, and activities. As Peace writes, "Material things are here for use, and anything you cannot relinquish when it has outlived its usefulness possesses you." She offers similar wisdom for living with the people in our lives, suggesting that a "live and let live" philosophy enables us to live in harmony with fellow humans.

The meditation for this chapter helps us realize how good we feel when we release unhealthy mental attachments by liberating our bodies as we think of these items. We will experience how good it feels to release clutching during specific thoughts. We realize we can better savor all the goodness in our lives without unhealthy attachments.

Finally, Peace tells us to relinquish all negative feelings. She writes, "If you live in the present moment, which is the only moment you have to live, you will be less apt to worry. If you realize that those who do mean things are psychologically ill, your feelings of anger will turn to feelings of pity. If you recognize that all of your inner hurts are caused by your own wrong actions or your own wrong reactions or your own wrong inaction, then you will stop hurting yourself." As you have been learning through the meditations, negative feelings restrict our energy. Peace is a perfect role model for this truth, demonstrating that when we release mental and physical negativity, well-being floods in to take its place.

Peace did not accomplish these four relinquishments quickly. It took her fifteen years, but her efforts had a huge payoff. As Peace writes:

So there were hills and valleys—lots of hills and valleys. Then in the midst of the struggle, there came a wonderful mountain-top experience, and for the first time I knew what inner peace was like. I felt a oneness—oneness with all my fellow human beings, oneness with all of creation. I have never felt really separate since. I could return again and again to this wonderful mountaintop, and then I could stay there for longer and longer periods of time, and just slip out occasionally.

Then came a wonderful morning when I woke up and knew that I would never have to descend again into the valley. I knew that for me, the struggle was over, that finally, I had succeeded in giving my life for finding inner peace. Again this is a point of no return; you can never go back into the struggle. The struggle is over now because you will do the right thing, and you don't need to be pushed into it.

I can vouch for Peace's discovery. The more I skillfully practice these relinquishments from the body level, my emotional baseline keeps increasing by practicing the highly skilled consciousness athlete meditations. I often find myself feeling exceptional joy during challenging moments, which I find both curious and delightful. I am confident that when you apply this same amount of earnest will, desire, and focus on your Happiness Athlete practice, you won't have to wait 15 years. These meditations, utilizing highly skilled biofeedback and subtle energy tools, will dramatically accelerate your efforts to release your body to propel it into joy.

Brother Lawrence's path is the final story I wish to share with you. His journey of complete surrender to a loving presence took him only ten years. Still, he continued surrendering into peace after that, his happiness continuing to escalate for an additional thirty years! By the end of his life, his joy was so unbounded, he actually had to strive to keep it quiet.

I have found myself in the same predicament occasionally and understand why he would do this. Unfortunately, our culture is not generally capable of graciously receiving happy people. I should warn you of that discovery. As your mood inevitably lifts after practicing this work, you will often find that you need to discover ways to channel the extra energy caused by your exuberance so as not to be abrasive to others. You will find yourself making different choices and starting to prefer your own company versus spending time with others who prefer to bond over misery.

Brother Lawrence often referred to himself in the third person, which gives us pause when considering how selflessness inspires happiness. For example, in this quote, Brother Lawrence describes himself: "for about thirty years his soul has been filled with joy and delight so continual, and sometimes so great, that he is forced to find ways to hide their appearing outwardly to others who may not understand."

Named Nicolas Herman, Brother Lawrence was born in 1614, to a family of humble means in France. To receive meals and a small stipend, he joined the time's war efforts and was severely wounded. His crippled body made him very clumsy, and in his own words, he was "a great awkward fellow who broke everything." Eventually, he became a lay-brother of the Carmelite Order and took the name of Brother Lawrence. Assigned to the kitchen until he suffered progressively worse gout, he was reassigned to a more manageable task, as sandal maker.

Brother Lawrence noticed the peace he felt when praying in the chapel and started to strive to feel that serenity at all times. He decided to dedicate every mundane task to God to relive the good feelings he experienced in the sanctuary. Every time his mind wandered, Brother Lawrence drew it back to God. He practiced the presence of God, similar to a musician practicing their instrument. At the ten year mark, he seemed to have reached the point similar to when Peace reached the point-of no-return to negativity.

During the following thirty years, he strived to further up-level his happiness through constant connection to God. Although he performed lowly work, his elevated consciousness became evident to all around him. Gradually, the humble sandal-maker's influence grew, not only among the poor but among the educated as well. Many learned people, religious, and ecclesiastics esteemed him. Because he did not want to disturb his connection to the Divine, he would offer only the most concise answers when called into administrative meetings, drenched with wisdom. Visitors, including politicians, would often seek guidance from Brother Lawrence. In conversations and letters, the knowledge he shared would later become the basis for the book, *The Practice of God's Presence* (which is found freely available online).

Like Peace Pilgrim and Lester Levinson, Brother Lawrence made his ascent into happiness through a relentless desire to experience something greater by applying highly skilled, gradual, consistent effort. Using his will, he cleansed his mind of negativity by conversing with the Divine over long periods. As he wrote, "To form a habit of conversing with God continually and referring all we do to Him, we must at first apply to Him with diligence. Then, after a little care, we would find his love inwardly draw us to Him without any difficulty . . . one does not become holy all at once."

We must remember Brother Lawrence's admonition that "one does not become holy all at once" if we are to be successful at the Happiness Athlete Program. There will be times after a defeat when you are frustrated, your energy is down, and you may start to doubt. You may say, "this stuff doesn't work." If that happens, get some rest, some food, meditate, and return to the work and keep at it! I guarantee that it is precisely at those moments that you are learning the most important lessons of all! As Brother Lawrence wrote, "if the mind is not sufficiently controlled and disciplined at our first engaging in devotion, it contracts certain bad habits of wandering and dissipation. These are difficult to overcome. The mind can draw us, even against our will, to worldly things." However, the more you honor these low times and treat them with a sacred presence and noble dignity, you will come to cherish the lessons you learn during the difficult times. You will discover that respecting those challenging days offers you the most extraordinary clarity, inspiring you to continue on your happiness journey to your inner freedom.

These three remarkable people each documented a profound phenomenon, demonstrating that we can elevate our consciousness into transcendent emotional states through the power of our own will. But they also illuminated another discovery for us: that there is no limit to the love, appreciation, and beauty we can all feel. Love is infinite, and only we ourselves are blocking it! "How high is up?" Lester was fond of saying. He recognized that up is only a relative term. There is no limit to up, as there is no limit to happiness. In fact, by letting go, Lester would burst into new levels of joy he had previously thought impossible. When he broke through to a higher state of love, he would say to himself, "This must be it. This must be the highest happiness anyone can feel. There can't be any more happiness than this." Then, after another round of releasing, his mood would lift even more. Exclaiming again, "This must be it! There can be no more love than this!" yet, he would later find himself basking in even more expansive levels of happiness. His happiness continued to elevate for thirty years until his death. I hope you are coming to realize this process is not rocket science. Elevated joy is merely an inevitable result of consistently and progressively releasing the body and energy field. That simple! All three of these people began their pursuits of happiness at extremely low points in their lives, as you may be doing right now. But keep at it! You GOT this!

In this chapter's meditation, we will explore this truth. We will experience how we are the only ones blocking our joy. We will also learn that love and happiness are limitless. Eventually, once we have done enough personal work, we will see clearly that the sky's the limit for our joy.

Notably, these remarkable individuals eventually

associated their profound happiness with a Divine intelligence that connects us. This may sound like a big stretch for agnostics, and I recognize that atheists are balking at the thought. I completely understand! I spent 13 years as an atheist, and it was the darkest period of my life. I still follow the atheist movement with great curiosity. Atheists who insist that God must be related to religion are missing the point. Associating God, exclusively with any religion, is an over-simplification, eclipsing a more significant, timeless, human experience. I agree with atheists that most of the world's atrocities have resulted from religion's limited perspective. However, based on my own experiences of the slower, higher, expanded brainwave states of consciousness, I must question anyone's conclusion that there is no higher order of connectedness. If you fall on the atheistic continuum, I respect your perspective and suggest substituting words such as light, spaciousness, emptiness, or expanded awareness for references to God or the Infinite. The meditation will still work nicely!

The concept of God has endured through millennia and across cultures because, integrally, we are wired to feel a connection to a loving intelligence that connects us all. When we train in slowing our brainwaves through meditation or EEG biofeedback, we become aware that we can access a larger field of intelligence. Unfortunately, to advance its own purposes of control, religion has overlaid over this hard-wiring of the soul. But this primary connection is indestructible. These meditations move us out of the dominant beta brainwaves that make us feel separate from this infinite intelligence. With a disciplined mind, we learn humility, experiencing a sincere connection with all things. We witness how reality shifts, according to brainwave dominance. Each set of brainwaves acts as a different filter to reality. We no longer exclusively trust and identify with every state we are in, once we recognize they are transient and learn the skills to navigate through them.

In this chapter's meditation, we will break out of our beta, analytical brainwaves that make us feel separate. We'll move into lower and slower brainwaves, enabling us to feel connected to something bigger. We will learn that feeling connected to the whole of the universe is a simple journey of surrendering the body to feel and sense something larger. We will start training ourselves to let go of little thoughts and lift into higher consciousness states. After a while, we will realize that even happy thoughts can be restricting. So, we will practice letting go of everything . . . and landing into higher and higher levels of lightness. Holding these states of consciousness, you will experience how sublime they are.

Now, your ego may say, "What?! Let go of everything? Even my job? My kids? My home?" To that, I respond, "if you want to feel light, alive and happy, yes." To be clear, as I said earlier, I am not telling you to sell everything and abandon your kids. What I mean is, stop the unhealthy drain on your energy concerning these things. What's exciting about this phenomenon is that when we skillfully let go of all that has been tugging on our energy system, we immediately lift into higher places. When we release the grip of our job, children, or spouse, we are more present when we are with them, which gives us a different set of healthier, responsive options. I realize this is counter-intuitive, but try it! You may be surprised at how your attachments were causing you to over-identify with things and eclipsing your ability to perceive potent solutions.

Let me help you reason this out, according to the most giant picture possible. You see, we are all on our way out of this world, eventually. Through this process, you will release everything in your life so that you can travel lightly to the other side. Fact. Let that sink in. This release that I speak of is part of the journey that we are already undergoing in our lives.

By disidentifying with life's challenges now instead of later, people see their lives with greater clarity, which fosters appropriate actions in all things now, with no regrets later. People who have near-death experiences (NDE's) often undergo a similar life review. From the perspective of the other side, they see their earthly life with exceptional clarity. Observing that their lives have gone off track, they return to their body, realizing they must make adjustments in their physical lives. Interestingly, after people have NDEs, they make incredible changes due to their new clarity about what is appropriate for their remaining days. When researchers wish to determine whether someone has had an actual NDE, they interview them to see whether their life has undergone a considerable transformation afterward. A highly "renovated life" is considered an indicator of a legitimate NDE.

People who experience NDEs also tell of the incredible love on the other side of the veil. Love beyond words. They come to understand that love is part of our infinite nature. When they return to their life here, they often recall this state of eternal love, realizing that life on earth is not all there is. When I read these accounts of such ineffable love, my attitude is always, "why wait?" I want to live from the state where I continually remember that I am eternal love now. I want to have that clarity now. I want to remember the grand journey I am on now, to live well, love well, and give well, now. I want to live a "no regret" life. Don't you? Every day, I strive to "stay awake at the wheel" and make decisions from this greater truth.

In the meditation for this chapter, I will be leading your nervous system into a more global release. In the prior meditations, we practiced how to release certain smaller portions of the body and energy field. By working in smaller areas, we received critical feedback about the mind's power to hone our increasing skill. However, in this meditation, we will move into an overall body release, toward universal love.

The changes in our bodies when we feel that love are significant. Our muscles relax, breathing slows, and blood flow rises to the surface of our skin. We can even say that love has a specific signature in the nervous system. We feel tenderness throughout our entire body. Through this softness, we eliminate feelings of separateness and start exploring our connection to others and infinite intelligence. Now that you know there is a curriculum for happiness that you determine through the quality of your own state of being, which determines your entire life's joy, are you willing to commit the mental focus toward releasing suffering in your body-mind? If you commit to this curriculum for happiness, I guarantee you will become happier. Once you understand that good feelings abound when we train our nervous system to lift into lightness, you will gain a profound understanding that will never leave you. You will become confident in this process. You learn you are indeed in charge of your happiness. You will even learn that applying these skills during struggles offers you exceptionally powerful opportunities to emerge into higher states of being.

Once you see the benefits of this work in your life, you will never turn back. As Peace said, "the struggle is over." You can't go back! You get addicted to feeling good. Nothing is worth selling out your exuberant vibe. You will become intolerant of feeling miserable, as other Consciousness Athletes and I have. Simple, but not always easy, this work takes dedication and a focused will. But the benefits mean you live life on *your* terms, in any circumstance.

I am excited to help you progress on your journey. This next meditation is where all of our singular efforts start to roll into a greater, more integrative experience. We will sculpt a new internal space for you, condition your body like an athlete's, and maintain buoyancy in daily life. As I have said, this kind of grace does not come cheap, but it is priceless! So put your time in, let yourself lift into lightness, and start to live from the sublime internal state that poets, mystics, and artists describe. As usual, I will ask you to note how you feel when you begin and how you feel at the end. Know that your state change occurred because of your willingness to discipline yourself to train like an athlete, in a skilled manner. You created this change, and it is up to you to continue conditioning yourself, to enhance this state of being. You have it in your power. I can vouch that it only gets better and sweeter, and it is worth every bit of effort! *You are worthy of your relentless and consistent effort!*

These experiences are only the beginning! You will start to experience what Brother Lawrence, Peace Pilgrim, and Lester Levinson discovered. However, you will progress more quickly than they did because you will be integrating powerful, proven biofeedback tools throughout your process.

Please practice this Expansive States for Higher Stakes - Letting Go Into Infinite Lightness mind-body exploration five times, before proceeding to the next chapter. Blow yourself away into bliss. Let yourself go. You've got this! Continue doing meditations with these advanced biofeedback skills. You, too, will get addicted to love and happiness because you will feel confident about how to create, sustain, and magnify them! This concrete confidence will occur because you will have the sweet satisfaction of knowing you earned them!

To access the *Expansive States for Higher Stakes— Letting Go Into Infinite Lightness* mind-body exploration, please visit Consciousness athletes.com/explorations

Enter the password: explore

Chapter Five Notes:
Conditioning Your Body For Happiness
By Transferring Consciousness Athlete Skills
into Daily Life

Please listen to the mind-body exploration for this chapter 5 times.

Always keep in mind, we learn to develop a greater capacity for happiness through three skills:

1. Coming into greater command of our nervous system.
2. Expanding our energy field.
3. Allowing ourselves to be carried into more buoyant lifted states.

To this end, practice calming your nervous system while becoming more aware of the space around your body. Practice maintaining a 360-degree awareness around the body, especially becoming aware of the area behind you.

In this chapter, we learned that positive emotions are infinite; we are the ones who block our joy through unhealthy ruminating patterns and accompanying unconscious physical tensions. When we learn how to let go of our physical restrictions and energy blocks skillfully, well-being automatically emerges. The more we become skilled at releasing ourselves from our emotional restrictions, we learn that we were responsible for our imprisonment. Simultaneously, we are grateful to recognize that we are not only capable of release, but we are responsible for our freedom.

To access the *Expansive States for Higher Stakes— Letting Go Into Infinite Lightness* mind-body exploration, please visit Consciousness athletes.com/explorations

Enter the password: explore

CHAPTER 6 - MULTIPLYING HAPPINESS BY SHARING IT

If you have read through the chapters and performed the five mind-body explorations five times, what significant progress you have made! You have learned how to boost your mood by transforming your internal environment significantly. That is no small accomplishment. Take a moment to appreciate your effort because few people will ever cultivate the level of internal discipline that you have already demonstrated. I hope you had fun gaining this level of mastery because in this chapter, you are going to learn how to gain even more gifts from your newly-acquired mental discipline.

By practicing the skills offered in this work, you are learning the art and science of intention. Maintaining intention requires us to sustain a strong and unwavering focus, especially in the face of challenge. You have been learning to make your mind steady and centered, to elicit significant internal change in the body, even when you may have wanted to give up or shut down emotionally. You are acquiring an impressive intentional grit! People suffering from excessive rumination, racing mind, and ADD struggle constantly because they have not learned how to strengthen their attention, as you have, to maintain their long term intentions.

Consider the phrase *"pay* attention!" That wording conveys the idea that your attention is so valuable; it has a monetary equivalent. Certainly, the e-commerce industry demonstrates this concept perfectly. The internet is continually vying for our attention because where we point our browser is most often where we spend our money. It is essential to realize that our attention is so precious, it should only be spent on things that are truly worth our focus.

In this day of streaming media and 24-hour news, we've become incredibly passive about how we direct our attention. Without much conscious thought, it is easy to surrender our mind for for hours to things like Netflix. While there is nothing wrong with doing this occasionally, is it possible that we are all getting a little too comfortable handing this precious commodity over to social media? Those precious hours of your life will never be returned. Are they worthy? The next time you reach for your device, take a moment to pause and ask, "What is best for me right now?" Reviewing the repetitive themes of a persistent crisis, which activates your nervous system's negativity bias? Or, rather, send your awareness deep within your cellular tissue to promote health, clarity, well-being, and wisdom? Just twenty minutes a day spent investing in the latter could create huge changes on a par with the butterfly's wings flapping in one hemisphere and causing a tsunami in the other.

As a Consciousness Athlete, you have been learning to rein in your attention in service to your greater internal healing intentions. If you are doing the mind-body explorations, I am 100% confident that you are already feeling better "seated" within yourself relative to when you started this book. You are becoming more discriminating about how you orient yourself in your world. I know this because of how the nervous system works. You can't do this work and not begin to feel more integrated and whole. It would be impossible—like going to the gym and lifting weights and *not* getting stronger.

So, the good news is that you have already been gaining increased mental strength. I hope I've made the process of retrieving your spirit back to your body so enjoyable that you didn't even notice you were doing attentional push-ups! Now that you have been gathering your energy back, we will learn how to use it to powerfully change your outer world as well. It is at this point that the Consciousness Athlete curriculum becomes really interesting!!

Remember back in 2006, when the groundbreaking film, *The Secret*, and eventually the book was released? It became a worldwide sensation. In it, Byrne writes that "the secret" is a law of the universe, taught since the beginning of time, described as "like attracts like." Another way to consider this "secret" is that what "we think about, we bring about." **The Secret** points out that our thoughts are more powerful than we've been taught, impacting the experiences, people, and circumstances we draw into our lives. Although still wildly successful, the film leaves out some gritty details about *how* to implement this law.

It is undeniable that our thoughts influence the quality of our lives. After all, we base our life choices, and the consequences or rewards they reap, on our belief systems. What is more often debated is whether a universal power contributes to these outcomes. *The Secret* asserts that there is a universal law of attraction that mirrors our thoughts back to us in the form of experience.The film's message is that if we focus our mind on what we want, we can have anything we want.

Simple, right? Well, what do you think? You have been becoming a Consciousness Athlete, so what have you learned about your focus? Are you able to maintain your focus 100% of the time in the face of a challenge? Are you able to stay true to your goals, even when the world is giving you discouraging feedback? Are you staying committed to making your dreams a reality?

If you are like most people, you would probably have to admit that you are not entirely consistent in focusing on your goals. As someone highly-versed in this field, sometimes I am still mentally slugging out issues to gain more clarity, as I learn to navigate deeper levels of consciousness. We often have to sift through emotional muck, to cull the clarity to remain steadfast in the face of obstacles. So, if there is, 1) a universal law that reflects back to us our mental and emotional states, and, 2) we are fluctuating internally, then, how could the universal mind reflect to us our one, preferred experience when we can't even mentally sustain it? It is at this point we come to understand just how fickle our minds can be. Whether we like to admit it or not, we often have severe deficits of psychological grit or staying power. For example, have you ever been so sure you were going to change your eating habits in the evening, but by the next day at 3:00 PM, you were already challenged, telling yourself, "I will start again tomorrow?" That is an entirely human response. However, that more disciplined "tomorrow" will never come until you gain enough command of your spirit to remain steadfast in the face of challenge. *A Course In Miracles* admonishes our fickle minds, "you are far too tolerant of mind wandering." After all, if like attracts like, and our minds are fluctuating back and forth between desired goals and destructive habits, how could this supposed universal law mirror back to us only our preferred result? That would not be a law. It would be an exception.

In the mind-body explorations of this book, you have been taking a front-row seat to observe the maneuvering of your mind. You are probably starting to sense that you have significantly different mindsets in different situations. We have been exploring your calm, deep mind, the part responsible for the creative, healing spaces you have been cultivating. We've also been discussing the unfocused mind, responsible for endless chatter, and the brutal inner critic who relentlessly assesses your past and future and often determines your unworthiness in the present. High beta brainwaves dominate this worried state of mind. This specific beta brainwave category, known as "beta three," is associated with significant stress, anxiety, paranoia, high energy, and increased arousal. When beta three brainwaves dominate, your mind may race, causing sleep disturbances (including nightmares), anger, aggression, anxiety, or impulsivity. Now, compare beta three brainwave feelings with the brainwaves you've been experiencing in the mind-body explorations—the lower brainwaves of alpha, theta, and delta. These inherently satisfying states of consciousness are often referred to as deep mind. In these quieter states, we are more loving, creative, and wise.

The wildly successful work of Dr. Joe Dispenza, and the Mind Mirror EEG body of work collected by Judith Pennington, suggest that when we are in these lower and slower brainwave states, we are more in tune with a sea of intelligent energy that surrounds our body. These pioneers suggest that we are tuned to receive information from the universal intelligence responsible for life itself when we have access to these states. Some may refer to this intelligence as God, the Great Spirit, Source, or Creator; others may refer to it as intuition or gut-knowing. It doesn't matter what label we use, but more and more research suggests that we are connected to a larger energetic field, connecting us all.

The more we condition our nervous systems to dive into deep mind, the more we realize we live in a greater field of intelligence that connects us all. We see a significant increase of delta brainwaves when people experience a profound connection with this universal field of intelligence. I have witnessed myself and others culling information from the universal field while in these lower brainwave states. Often, I have been in the lower brainwaves of deep mind and plucked information from the universal intelligent mind that I did not have access to in ordinary consciousness. Often, when I finish my meditation, I go right to the internet to check on the validity of what I downloaded. I am nothing special at this, as I have witnessed the same phenomenon hundreds of times in my clients and groups. When this starts to occur for you—and it will if you keep practicing, if it hasn't already—you may choose to start committing even more deeply to your meditation practice. The mysteries are simply too enticing to ignore!

It is a well-known secret among devoted meditators that the more we meditate, the more synchronicities or coincidences occur in our lives. The Merriam-Webster dictionary defines synchronicities as "the coincidental occurrence of events and especially psychic events (such as similar thoughts in widely separated persons or a mental image of an unexpected event before it happens) that seem related but are not explained by conventional mechanisms of causality." The concept of synchronicities as having more significance than merely "random coincidence" was developed in the work of psychologist, C. G. Jung. Dedicated meditators such as internationally-known author, Dr. Deepak Chopra, and founding scientist of the opiate receptor, Dr. Candace Pert, have observed that the more we meditate, the more synchronicities we experience. Chopra and Pert attribute a large part of their own enormous personal success to meditation and have suggested that they attracted their success through their practice of expanding their consciousness. I remember Pert once saying, "Did I discover the opiate receptor or did I create the opiate receptor?" She was implying that through her intentions, incessant questioning, and reasoning that there must be an opiate receptor in the body, she may have beckoned forth the opiate receptor from this sea of intelligence that connects us all.

I have been a dedicated meditator for over twenty-five years. Through these experiences, I have learned that there is a wider "wisdom thread" running through my life, but I can see it most clearly when I remain near my center, and anchored in my lower brainwaves. It has taken me a long time to realize that the most powerful place I can be is on my meditation cushion, snuggling up to Infinite. The more I meditate and practice becoming a pure vessel for this field of intelligence, the more I trust my life. I am often told that I have "perfect timing," and synchronicities have become common. Meditation primes me to work in accordance with this wisdom that is far greater than my own.

For the Law of Attraction to work for us, we need to cultivate the discipline of a stilled mind so that we can sense this benevolent intelligence, to develop a relationship with it. Would you ever walk up to someone on the street and give them the keys to your car? Of course not. You would only do that with friends and family. People with whom you have a relationship. It's the same with this field of intelligence that connects us all: before we can trust it with the big situations in our lives, we need to cultivate a relationship with it through the problems in our lives. Through small miracles, we gain greater confidence to maintain the relationship and turn to it for help with the more significant concerns. While doing the Consciousness Athlete mind-body explorations, the great news is that you have already been cultivating this relationship with something larger than yourself. You may have already begun noticing subtle changes in your environment as you've been practicing these skills.

In the mind-body explorations, you've been harnessing your attention to serve your intentions for healing, wholeness, and happiness. In this context, we are defining intention as your goal, purpose, or plan. Skilled sitters use the lower brainwaves cultivated in meditation to set their intentions. For Law of Attraction to work in your best interests, you need to have an overall concentrated intention, even when your life is in chaos and uncertainty. Meditation gives us the practical training for staying steady during times of adversity.

Advanced meditators and intenders know that

what appear to be obstacles are opportunities for obtaining greater clarity. We also understand that anything in our psyche that is not congruent with our goal needs to be cleansed and released before we can manifest, which is why our meditation practice is so invaluable. At the beginning of working with intention, it can feel really rocky. In fact, people often get very frustrated by how much needs to be cleared before the goal can manifest. As far as I am concerned, learning to hold your mind's focus, especially in the body, is the best skill you could pursue to cultivate the mental discipline required for success with the Law of Attraction. Navigating through the storms of life, applying the skills that you have been acquiring, you'll gain a deeper understanding of what is required to thrive.

In this chapter, we will combine all that we have learned so far—focusing the mind for maximal impact, anchoring the mind in the tan tien, opening the heart, releasing emotional addictions, and letting go into lightness—to serve the grander intentions for your entire life. We will learn how to employ these powerful, beautiful skills you've been honing, putting them in greater service for yourself and the world. You've been practicing calibrating your mind and body toward wholeness and expanding your energy field into your surroundings. We will now begin working on expanding your consciousness, even more, to facilitate experiencing greater peace, joy, and abundance.

Have you ever been in your car at a stoplight, and subconsciously, you find your head turning? When you turn your head, you suddenly find yourself looking eye-to-eye with someone who's been staring at you? Rupert Sheldrake, biologist, author, and recognized thought leader, has been exploring this phenomenon for over twenty-five years. He refers to it as the "sense of being stared at." He found that 74% of men and 81% of women report that they have experienced this sense. Interestingly, significantly more women (88%) compared to men (71%) said they had found they could stare at others and make them turn around. Maybe now that you've experienced the power of your own focused mind in your body, you understand how this could be possible. As we said in the first chapter, your mind has impact! Be careful with it, especially since you have been honing your mental discipline! Now we'll start using your new skills—that have caused powerful changes in your body—to create powerful changes in your external world.

A famous research study, known as the Love study, demonstrates our mind has impact outside of the body. In this study, researchers observed 31 married couples who were divided into three groups. One was a healthy control group, where both spouses were healthy. The other two groups included one spouse who had cancer. One of these groups had received training in sending compassionate intention to their spouse, and the other group did not receive any training. Both spouses in all of the groups were connected to biofeedback instrumentation, which measured physiological variables such as skin conductance, heart rate, blood flow, and respiration. Only one spouse was looking at a TV screen image of their spouse in another electromagnetically-shielded room. The other spouse (specifically the sick spouse in the couples with cancer) was in another room, nicely tucked into a recliner with a camera recording them. The spouse in the room with the TV screen was instructed to send their spouse loving, healing intentions when they randomly saw their spouse appear on the screen.

The biofeedback measurements revealed that sending intentions generates palpable, measurable energy. The nervous system response of the receivers tracked the sender's physiological response. When the sender sent healing intention, the spouse's body became measurably activated, as evidenced by synchronized results in skin conductance rate, blood flow, and respiration. Interestingly, the most prolonged pattern occurred among the cancer patients whose partners had been trained in compassionate intention, which revealed a "training effect."

Those trained to send loving intentions had more measurable results than those who did not. As we have been learning, the more we practice using intention, the better measurable results we obtain.

Another group of intentional studies I like to refer to are the prayer studies for plants. I like plant prayer research because sending intentions to plants and measuring changes is much easier than sending intentions to people. I often quip that you will get better results praying for your plants than praying for your spouse because plants won't resist your intentions! If you pray for plants to grow taller and stronger, research suggests they actually listen. Lynne McTaggart, the world's leading expert on intention, and psychologist Dr. Gary Schwartz, director of the Center for Advances in Consciousness and Health at the University of Arizona, performed an experiment demonstrating the power of human intentions on plants through their geranium leaf experiments. In these experiments, they wanted to measure whether people could cause an increase in the number of biophotons, or light, that geranium leaves emitted. Biophoton emission is the spontaneous emission of ultra-weak light from all living systems, including humans. By flipping a coin, the audience chose one of two identical leaves, poked with 16 holes. McTaggart asked them to send intention for ten minutes to the selected leaf and invite it to "glow and glow" with light. The scientists were not told which leaf was chosen before performing the post-experiment calculations. Dr. Schwartz revealed that the changes in the light emissions of the leaf given the glowing intention were so strong, the light could be seen readily in the digital images created by CCD cameras. Numerically, the increased biophoton effect was statistically highly significant.

Dozens of other plant and seed studies demonstrate this reliable effect of human intention on simple organisms. When it comes to humans, prayer and intentional studies become less definitive. As you have learned about yourself, humans are far more complex creatures who have learned the tenacity of clinging to their emotional addictions, which makes them far less influenced by external intentions. The plant research confirms that human intentions definitely yield external results. However, over time, some reliable patterns are emerging that suggest humans can influence each other over distance. For instance, the Transcendental Meditation organization has repeatedly demonstrated that when a relatively small number of trained meditators are gathered in an area to meditate to increase the peace, a reduction of violence is observed in that local geographic area. A 2016 study published in *SAGE Open,* titled, "Societal Violence and Collective Consciousness: Reduction of U.S. Homicide and Urban Violent Crime Rates," documented that group practice of Transcendental Meditation was linked with decreased homicides and violent crime in the US, during the 2007-2010 study period. Researchers hypothesized that relatively few people meditating together would create a nationwide positive effect. From January 2007 through 2010, over 1,725 participants gathered to practice group Transcendental Meditation at Maharishi University of Management in Fairfield, Iowa. Researchers found an 18.5% drop in violent crime nationwide at the end of the study. Statistical and independent analyses showed the rising trend of US homicides during 2001-2006 was reversed during the 2007-2010 study period. Other variables were ruled out, such as the economy, demographics, and law enforcement.

Lead author, Dr. Michael Dillbeck commented on these astonishing results, saying, "I understand it's a new hypothesis in the social sciences that meditation could have a stress-reducing and coherence-creating effect in society. "But such research is increasingly suggesting that there's a field effect of consciousness. If you get a large enough group together practicing this technique to experience the field quality of consciousness, these extended 'field-like' effects are expressed in society."

If you are a curious skeptic like me, you may have questions such as, "how can you definitely link those positive societal measurements to be the result of *that* group's meditations?" I understand your hesitation to accept this conclusion. I wanted to test this myself, so my nonprofit, NUMINOUS, created an outreach branch, called the Global Peaceful Cities Project. Through this initiative, I wanted to give cities the opportunity to gather to perform meditation peace research studies in their own home town, to test group meditation's efficacy on a smaller scale.

By scaling the research down to the neighborhood level, we could isolate influencing variables much more effectively. To date, we have performed two studies that revealed significant results. The first, completed in 2018, demonstrated a 25% reduction of violent crime in a neighborhood in Schenectady, NY. The second study revealed a 30% reduction of crime in Albany, NY.

Dr. Karina Reinhold, State University of New York at Albany Professor of Mathematics and Statistics, and I are prepared to help others take this work into their cities. My highest hope is that readers of my books consider organizing their own neighborhood peace projects. Dr. Reinhold and I can support you in your peace project endeavors. Our years of experimenting through trial and error have shown that we need approximately 1% of the geographic area's population meditating for peace to obtain a measurable result. Remarkably, not all of the meditators have to be in the geographic area that is being measured.

People participate in our experiments from all over the world. If you are passionate about teaching people how to use meditation to promote peace in your area, we will invite the people on our list to send intentions for peace to your area as well. Please reach out to us if you are interested in performing a peace project in your neighborhood.

I have worked hard to overcome many complex obstacles in order to provide this opportunity for non-researchers who are passionate about improving their communities to participate in our research, because I am passionate about helping people understand the power of their own minds to change the world. To this end, in the mind-body exploration for this chapter, I will be teaching you how to focus your intention to positively influence challenging situations in your life. We will learn to combine all of the skills that we have been practicing to not only improve your life but also the lives of others, as well. We will open our hearts, connect to infinite love, and practice expanding our consciousness to people and situations we would like to influence positively. We will send intentions for the "highest and best for all concerned" to facilitate supportive change.

The Consciousness Athletes and I have often been delighted to find that when intentions are sent for the collective good of everyone involved in a situation, the field of infinite consciousness has a way of calculating all the variables, often including those that are hidden, and elegantly yielding an outcome that serves everyone. We have been able to track our progress by sharing our results when we come together once a month. For each class in the Consciousness Athlete program, I present a new expanding consciousness skill and create a meditation that helps people practice coming into command of their nervous system while expanding their subtle energy field. I leave time in the meditation for two extra steps. First, I invite them to use their new skill to facilitate sending loving intentions to difficult situations in their own lives, and then, I have them use the same skill to support someone else in the class. I allow plenty of time for people to share how their intentions have been making positive impacts in their lives. When we hear of the successes that people experience over time, we learn to be patient. We develop a deep abiding trust in the process, even when our personal intentions may not appear to be manifesting.

It can be discouraging when we can't see immediate external results from our intentions. But remember, we are training like athletes to condition the body for high performance. A dedicated athlete would not become discouraged and quit after just a week. An athlete learns how to train for the long haul. Consciousness Athletes become disciplined to cultivate the tenacity of mind required to maintain their intentions over time, especially in the face of significant obstacles and adversity. They are capable of such steadfastness because they live from the understanding that their intentions are always being transmitted into the field of consciousness that connects us all. Working with a group, hearing about others' successes while you may be struggling gives you the inspiration and fortitude to continue during challenging times.

During each class, I work to help people refine their intentions for the greatest impact. The details for sending powerful constructive intentions could fill another book which I may feel called to write in the future. I can share these distilled details in my advanced classes, however, for our purposes in this chapter, just remember: maintaining the highest and best intentions for all will always steer you in the correct direction. The Universe has a way of calculating the needs of everyone involved for their maximum evolution.

We strive to maintain impeccable integrity with our intentions. Because we know how intentions influence our lives, we are frequently careful to release any negativity that could hamper our progress. Because Consciousness Athletes know that what they send out in the world will return to them; they would never wish bad outcomes for anyone. You will find that only wishing the highest and best for all, even and especially for people who challenge you, is an ennobling skill-set, offering rare opportunities for the cultivation of both integrity and dignity. You will come to like and respect yourself more through this process. We don't seem to experience our inherent dignity until it is challenged. I guarantee that you will like and respect yourself more by wishing goodwill for all others.

To help manage all of the unknown elements of sending intentions, I suggest you use light in meditation. Focusing light is the single most crucial tool for people starting in this work. Virtually all of the religious traditions speak of humans as beacons of light. As shown in the glowing leaf experiment, discussed earlier in this chapter, current science has determined that all living organisms emit tiny packages of light, called biophotons. A prominent focus in biophoton emissions research is how they transmit messages throughout an organism's cells. For example, when a green bean is cut in two, small photons travel back and forth between each piece! Isn't that interesting?

While a full discussion of biophotons is beyond the scope of this book, you may notice that when I use light in the meditation, your intentional effort becomes more substantial. I have heard that light is one of the universe's building blocks, and I believe it. The strength and resilience people gain by working with light changes the trajectory of their lives. I suggest you start playing with it as much as possible, such as imagining light between the hearts involved or feeling your chest swell with light. Just imagining light wakes up our entire brain. The more people work with light in their meditations, the more impact the meditations yield. I was literally jarred in my seat when I was working with a pillar of light one day. It was so intense, palpable, significant, I shifted in my seat to accommodated it as it touched me. Truth be told, I often feel "in love" with light daily, and often wake up at night being bathed in light, especially during my darkest times. I don't know what it means exactly, but it has become my constant companion. I am so *grateful* I have a beautiful place to park my mind during scary times. I wouldn't want to live on this planet during these dark and challenging times without access to this perpetually available presence. Many Coherence Athletes have their own powerful experiences with light as well.

After we clear dense energies in our system, we are all able to feel light's effects. Even if you are not at the point where you feel light as physically impactful, light still symbolizes illumination and understanding, something we can all appreciate.

There has been another consistent thread in our Global Peaceful Cities Project. Over the years, we have observed a phenomenon so consistent, we finally measured its robust results. After participating in peace projects, people became happy—substantially more happy! It was evident in the comments people wrote and the cards we received. We repeatedly witnessed a wave of creativity occur in participants' lives when the peace projects were completed. People often start pursuing endeavors that they have been stifling for years. I asked our lead researcher, Dr. Karina Reinhold to help us measure these enormous changes in happiness. The results could be considered astonishing, but they weren't to us because we had witnessed this phenomenon many times. Our 2018 study calculated that people who participated in our peace projects for only eight days experienced a whopping 84% increase in happiness! The following year, people experienced a 68% increase. I suspect the lower score was due to website issues we were experiencing at the time. Either way, would you care to experience a 68% or 84% relative increase in happiness in eight days from today? Who wouldn't? This boost in mood is *hugely* significant.

I hope that after reading this book and performing the accompanying mind-body explorations, you are not surprised at these results, either. Simply put, we can't skillfully focus our awareness on lightening our heart and expanding our energy field to send intentions for peace and goodness to others, and *not* feel happier, correct? Again, that would be like lifting weights repeatedly and not getting stronger. That would be impossible, correct? It's the same principle with this work: you can't skillfully practice these methods and remain the same as you were before. It would be impossible.

Again, I will not ask that you accept my word for any of this. I am asking you to perform the mind-body exploration for this chapter, to experience this uplift yourself! This mind-body exploration will draw on all the internal intentional skills you have been learning to enhance and uplift not only your body but your entire life. By expanding our point of awareness, and sending loving intentions, we will learn how this work changes our experience of everything, especially our challenges! Be sure to notice the greater strength in your spirit and spring in your step after finishing this meditation. Those tangible shifts are repeatable, demonstrating that you are doing the work correctly.

Just like any athlete, you have to continue opening and expanding to maintain your buoyant mood because you will lose your conditioning if you don't. However, the benefit is that you always gain *immediate* results! You will soon become addicted to feeling good, gaining the understanding that *nothing* is worth giving up your levity. Light becomes your home you never want to leave. You experience the benefit of becoming a citizen of the field of loving consciousness that surrounds you. You yearn for everyone to learn about their birthright to feel fabulous, which may even inspire you to create your own peace project or offer your genius to uplift the world around you, as your creativity flares. When we are creative, we spiral upward towards pure emotional freedom and become even closer to infinite love. The valleys we experience become merely the foot of the next mountain we will conquer.

You have learned the game of life, and you are playing it well. You are seizing your power and refusing to submit it to any tragedy. No person, situation, or crisis, can rob you of the skills you have learned to fall up! Life finally becomes the magical, meaningful ride it is supposed to be. Best of all, you know you have conditioned your mind and body to reach these heights, so you know how to stay there and expand into it more. The best part is that you have also learned that love and joy are infinite. You have earned the skills to be a rare explorer of human consciousness to experience states of beauty available to everyone. But, tragically, these states are currently out of reach for most people only due to lack of training. Because you feel so good and you know exactly how you got there, all you want to do is help everyone get there as well, as I am doing now.

To find the *Multiplying Happiness By Sharing It* exploration, please visit ConsciousnessAthletes.com/explorations

Enter the password: explore

Chapter Six Notes:
Conditioning Your Body For Happiness
By Transferring Consciousness Athlete Skills
into Daily Life

Please perform the mind-body exploration, *Multiplying Happiness By Sharing It,* for this chapter 5 times.

When you find yourself worrying about your life, start to change these mental habits. Try bathing the situation in love and light.

See just how big you can expand the subtle energy field of your heart area, widen your energy field, and then widen your awareness into your city, state, country and eventually around the globe. Notice how the more you widen your awareness, the more at peace you feel.

Connect the hearts of everyone involved through love and light, setting the intention for the highest and best for all concerned.

Notice how good it feels to dissolve the personal ego and merge with the field of benevolent intelligence surrounding you.

Please   visit consciousnessathletes.com/explorations

Enter the password: Explore

EPILOGUE - AN INVITATION

I feel passionate about increasing my knowledge base, gaining greater command of my nervous system, expanding my subtle energy field, and enjoying ever more lifted states of consciousness. Aside from raising my children, I have placed increasing my personal consciousness skills above virtually all worldly concerns. In future books, I will describe why I prioritize this focus in ways that would raise eyebrows among the more conventional.

My enjoyment of exploring new vistas and dislike of writing delayed this book: documenting my life's work in a book seemed like a tedious endeavor. I knew it was my challenge to find a way to systematize the process. I am fully aware that this work could appear trite to the uninitiated. Consciousness Athlete experiences are far outliers to everyday experiences. I know that people are unable to grasp the work unless they have done such work. Simply put, these or similar steps must be pursued until basic mastery is acquired before their gifts are revealed. This kind of grace does not come cheap, but success is imminent with dedication. It is to this end that I finally delineated the steps to ensure your success.

As an avid explorer of the unknown of consciousness, I'm having great fun on my journey, along with my advanced Consciousness Athletes. I'm incredibly blessed by their company. My students are some of my greatest teachers. Our history of discovering consciousness together allows us to share references to large bodies of experiences in just a sentence or two! Among the many memorable gifts and insights my students have offered, the most important is that they taught me there are objective signposts within this vague field of consciousness that can be seen and experienced by all! Because I have enjoyed working with them so much, I have felt reticent about starting new classes. However, now that I've documented these fundamental Consciousness Athlete skills, I am excited. I've created an opportunity for more people to follow my step-by-step program, allowing them to expand consciousness and finally live from more pleasant states of well-being. Now, I am very much looking forward to teaching new students again.

If you find you want to continue gaining the benefits of pursuing the Consciousness Athlete work in a more structured approach, I am creating several opportunities to continue to learn within a formal Consciousness Athlete curriculum. Periodically, I will offer a four-month Consciousness Athlete program. Having studied with some of the greatest healers of our time, both in the states and abroad, I have assembled this program by cherry-picking the best practices I have cultivated over 25 years. You have experienced a sample of such content in this book. There is so much ground to cover. The journey to expanding consciousness could feel overwhelming, but I make each step of the way manageable, offering specific feedback to help accelerate your results. I confidently teach with the secured end goal in mind because I want to inspire you that are worthy of your own effort. You got this! Throughout this work, you will come to a greater understanding of the benefits of living life as a Consciousness Athlete. As I've emphasized repeatedly in this book, your end goal is athletically conditioning your nervous system for heightened consciousness.

However, I have included two more aspects in the curriculum that I could not add in this book due to logistical limitations. These elements can dramatically accelerate your trajectory when they are integrated within your journey. First, in the four-month program, you have the opportunity to share your personal goals while receiving skilled intentional coaching from the rest of the Consciousness Athlete class and me. Take that in for a moment. It is a unique and incredibly rare opportunity. Each class you can enter your name on the master spreadsheet, so you will receive support to achieve your goals from the powerful, skilled intentions of fellow *trained* students!

As we have learned, research demonstrates that intention has a "training effect." It is best to receive intentions from people who are trained. Since intentions are powerful, you want to be sure people sending intentions your way are sending them correctly! You will be confident that your fellow students will "have your back!" My students often joke that they know when it is their day to receive intentions, because they can feel the "ju ju," or juicy energy, of the increased flow of energy in their lives that day. That increase in energy is often just what they need to "fall up" into a new state of being.

The second powerful aspect of this course, one you will not see offered in many programs, is that I often allow time for group communication. The wisdom that comes from the participants, who have been cleansing their consciousness, is often appropriately insightful, revealing greater wisdom. You may meet some of your newest, closest friends in our classes! We consider our time together a rare and precious gift. A student once expressed the importance of this, saying, "Frank and I could not make it to class...and we were truly pained by that."

I am also creating a website, sponsored by my nonprofit interfaith organization, Numinous, that will continue to support your consciousness expansion. This website will be a resource for a small monthly fee to help you continue your consciousness expansion studies through a proven system. A cornerstone of the website will be the meditation library, offering an array of meditations created to meet Consciousness Athletes' advanced skill. These meditations are designed to guide you into greater physical mastery of your nervous system while simultaneously expanding your subtle energy field. Each mind-body exploration is expressly created to offer you transferable life skills, successfully implementing intentional skills in your daily life. Additionally, most meditations build in time for sending intentions not only to your life but to the lives of people you care about and love. The Consciousness Athlete website will provide you with the daily training and encouragement needed to keep conditioning yourself to sustain lifted states of consciousness.

My advanced students have taught me the immense benefits of sharing this work. We are all each other's research experiments, as we observe the positive impact of the Consciousness Athlete curriculum on us all. I am deeply indebted to them because people can only vouch for the Consciousness Athlete curriculum's benefits *after* they have dedicated time to practice the work. Their endorsements do not come from acquiring only intellectual understandings. Instead, their support is based on their experiences gleaned after learning how to skillfully lead the body's nervous system into a deep mind. Lacking these experiences as a reference point, these concepts could sound like "New Age nonsense" to the uninitiated.

For this reason I am creating a fee-based membership site, where I can offer feedback, wisdom, and advice, encouragement solely to those who are dedicated and earnest in their heightened consciousness pursuits. Because you have read this book and have practiced all the mind-body explorations, I can speak to you at a more advanced level than the general public. Working purely with dedicated explorers, we will all learn from each other and expand together. I will encourage interactions between students and personally answer as many questions as possible.

We all learn the most when Consciousness Athletes ask questions. These spontaneous exchanges often set the stage for surprising and delightful discoveries. The online community forum will support our endeavors to eliminate our dense energies to live from more lighthearted spaces.

Before deciding whether you want to continue working with the Consciousness Athletes, let's take a moment to integrate your learning from this book. We began our journey together by experiencing the stark difference between having your mind's awareness anchored in your body, versus ruminating without boundaries. You were able to objectively feel the vertical line, differentiating between your right and left side, when you anchored your mind in only your right side. You realized the pleasure of being anchored in your body, even though only on the right. Remember my question: "how much better would you feel in life if you learned to remain anchored in your body at all times?"

In chapter two, you learned about anchoring your mind in your tan tien, holding your power in your body, and not hemorrhaging it to external situations or substances. You practiced how to maintain the detached, resourceful state of mind of being anchored in your tan tien, which offers us a far broader range of options than we possess while in the stress response. We learned how to foster unwavering resilience by merely finding a new place in our body.

We learned how to manage our heart like a garden in chapter three by weeding it of resentments and watering it with love, beauty, and appreciation.

We also learned that we can't feel happy without cultivating a light heart, and we learned to be "happy for no good reason."

In chapter four, we learned what I believe is one of the most important skills, one that almost no one knows. This is the pivotal skill of locating your emotional addiction in your body, and removing it with precision, allowing your negative moods to lift, freed from the weight of a constellation of unresolved, dense energy.

Chapter five discussed how to expand our being states for higher stakes by letting go into lightness. This is my favorite chapter because it offers us a logical and predictable framework for our curriculum. Brother Lawrence, Peace Pilgrim, and Lester Levenson each left us written work documenting their journey into divinely-inspired consciousness. If you have been performing the mind-body explorations, what they say makes total sense, right? Let's all set an intention to let go of the denser energies in our field, so we can automatically lift upward. When we release heaviness, our spirit lifts with directed power, similar to how a buoy shoots up out of the water after being held under with resistance for so long.

In the final chapter, we learned how to use our newly-cultured mental discipline to send intentions for peace and happiness to our lives and the lives of others. We learned that our non-local mind can change situations outside of space and time. Take a moment and appreciate how far you have come! You have traversed to places that few people have had the opportunity to explore. You were willing to invest in your spirit, to find this gorgeousness within you that was there all along! Kudos to you! So, what is next for you? You may want to consider joining the Consciousness Athlete community to accelerate your future results.

There is a truth regarding all living systems: if we are not growing, we are dying. Nature never stays the same. So, understand that as good as you feel now, you will lose some of your gains if you stop practicing. However, if you keep coming into command of your nervous system and expanding your energy field through Consciousness Athlete skills, you will build your capacity to sustain joy. Love is Infinite! Good feelings will abound in your life. So, what is your choice? I hope you continue exploring and cleansing your energy field and coming into greater command of your nervous system. This work blesses every aspect of your life. And, eventually, your death as well. When your body has decided it has served its full use, you will already have the understanding that at death, you are merely expanding into ineffable love. You are worthy of your loving attention to pursue the most important journey of your life. By conditioning your body like an athlete to sustain heightened states of consciousness, you will have earned your well-being. No one can rob you of your joy. You will be falling up from now on.

Godspeed,

Bethany